ALIVE
with
TOMORROW'S
MEDICINE

Kristy Moore Hernandez

How I Live a Happy, Healthy, Pain Free Life
with
Chemical Intolerance,
Environmental Illness,
and
Multiple Chemical Sensitivity

<u>DEDICATION</u>

I dedicate this book to all seekers of wellness and truth. May your search be fulfilled and the suffering be over.

TABLE OF CONTENTS

iv

<u>Preface</u>

"Everything is determined... by forces over which we have no control. It is determined for the insect as well as the star. Human beings, vegetables, or cosmic dust- we all dance to a mysterious tune, intoned in the distance by an invisible piper."
~Albert Einstein~

This is the book I was looking for thirty years ago. A book that couldn't be found because it had not yet been written. Twenty years later I would search in vain once again for this book. Three years ago I had an epiphany; I was the one to write the book.

How to Use this Book

Enclosed within these pages is my own unique odyssey from sickness to health. I have laid out the book in four sections.

Part One:
The Problem

Part One includes what I have discovered as a result of years of research. It also explains why doctors and health care providers are challenged with diagnoses and treatment of these conditions.

Part Two:
The Experience

Part Two is where I share how I walked (sometimes crawled) away from chemical dangers and how I was guided to a new foundation of health. My reward was recovering my most precious possession... good health.

Part Three:
The Solutions

Part Three focuses on what worked for me. What I did, and how I did it. I will give you a new language of wellness and lay out a new foundation for true vibrant health, where homeostasis is reached. I will guide you through the solutions that helped me regain my life back: my return to *homeostasis*. This is where you will learn another way to transform the pain and symptoms of Multiple Chemical Sensitivities (MCS), Chemical Intolerance (CI),

Environmental Illness (EI), and Idiopathic Environmental Intolerance (IEI).

Part Four:
The Resources

Part Four of the book includes my sources, web addresses, a bibliography, MSDS information, sources for products that assisted me in my recovery and books that helped form my attitude for healing.

<u>**Acknowledgments**</u>

Books don't just happen. It takes a dedicated mind to write a book and a critical mind for details to edit one. In my case it took a team of superheroes, called editors, Kara Aitken, Kim Johnson, and Daya Callan, for they each took my mess of words, years of research, and experiences and with each of their unique contributions helped me bring forth from the chaos, the truth as I humbly know it. Their help was invaluable in explaining how I took thirty-three years of surviving with chemicals and crafted my life into the peaceful place I am today. With their kind encouragement, patience and skills a book is brought forth that is a witness, a testament to the truth that Tomorrow's Medicines work.

Marvis Moore, Eileen Seitz, and Susan Hally, thank you for cheering me on, by reading, and helping with polishing my message. Heather Holmes, thank you for sharing generously all you learned along your own healing path. Judy Adam, Barbara Graham and Victoria Rose, thank you for being here now.

To my family and friends I want to acknowledge your love and support and express how grateful I am to have you all in my life. Thank you Kim Kisling for being a true friend who was present and listened as I came face to face with my personal truth through the decades.

Thank you husband, son and daughter. It has been a rough ride on a hard road and I appreciate your sacrifice, support and love. I know you haven't had a life like others, but look on the bright side, you haven't had a life like others!

PART ONE:

The Problem

This section is dedicated to a brief explanation of the problem that is hurting us all.

<u>INTRODUCTION</u>

"In matters concerning truth and justice there can be no distinction between big problems and small; for the general principles which determine the conduct of men are indivisible. Whoever is careless with the truth in small matters cannot be trusted in important affairs."
~Albert Einstein~

If you've picked up this book, chances are you or someone you love has been sick and suffering for a very long time without an adequate explanation as to why. Do you have an underlying sense that something is not right but your medical tests are normal? Are your doctors unable to find a medical reason or a diagnosis for your failing health? Do you desperately want to understand why your body is failing? Are you feeling alone and hopeless? Are you or a loved one desperate for relief? ***Are you terrified of dying without an answer as to why you are so sick?***

I know I was.

I've spent many years of my life sick. My doctors could not offer a cure for my many varied ailments. I was desperate to be relieved of constant headaches, fatigue, lowered immune response, digestive stress, menstrual madness, skin issues, and liver dysfunction that troubled me for decades.

I finally found relief.

I'm excited to share my journey and my solutions with you in hopes that you can find relief as well. If you or a loved one relate to any of the above issues, it's very possible that you may be dealing with:
- Multiple Chemical Sensitivities (MCS)
- Chemical Intolerance (CI)

4

- Environmental Illness (EI)
- Idiopathic Environmental Intolerance (IEI)

You may also be searching for answers to other labels and diagnoses such as:

- Chronic Fatigue Syndrome
- Fibromyalgia
- Gulf War Syndrome
- Methylenetetrahydrofolate Reductase (MTHFR)
- Premenstrual Syndrome (PMS)
- Premenstrual Dysphoric Disorder (PMDD)
- Stress

Perhaps you've been labeled with a psychosis such as:

- Anxiety
- Chemophobia
- Depression
- Hypochondria
- Obsessive Compulsive Disorder

Some of you may have been searching years for relief from:

- 20th Century Disease
- Allergies
- Cerebral Allergy
- Chemical Hypersensitivity Syndrome
- Dystonia
- Food Intolerance or Sensitivities
- Inflammation
- Pain
- Premature Aging
- Sick Building Syndrome
- Total Allergy Syndrome
- Universal Allergy

How do all of these diagnoses and illnesses relate? Based on my research and personal experiences, I declare that these are all branches of the same tree, the same malady, with many different names and manifestations, but with the same roots - **chemical intolerance**.

Enclosed within these pages is my own unique odyssey from sickness to health. Within the four parts to my book I'm going to communicate with you the truth of my observations and experiences with chemicals, the symptoms of chemicals and how some health conditions relate to a big chemical picture. I'm also excited to share how it was possible for me to escape these ailments and live a full, healthy life without suffering!

Many years ago I set out onto an unbeaten path searching for a way to return to health. In this book I will share with you everything I've learned, but most importantly I will show you exactly what worked for me. I am living proof that this way works. I am a testament that even with dire circumstances a person can recover and return to health with Tomorrow's Medicine.

If you are seeking the keys to unlock the secrets of true wellness, may this book be your saving grace and guide through the storm of confusion to get to the truth. May my story help you see that **you are not alone**.

Let's begin this journey by starting off with some basic information.

Defining MCS, CI, EI, IEI
Oh My! I'm Still SIC!

What is Multiple Chemical Sensitivity (MCS)? Multiple Chemical Sensitivities or MCS, is defined as an individual who reacts with sensitivity to different chemicals such as gasoline, perfume, and cleaning products. An individual with MCS will react with undefined symptoms to one, some, or all of these chemicals. When others are exposed to the same chemicals, they may experience different symptoms or no symptoms at all for several years. However, there are people who *do not know* that they're symptomatic and have conditions such as swollen arms and legs. A person may think it's simply a lack of exercise – a concept society has imposed upon them. Yet the enlarged extremities may very well be due to a reaction to chemicals and once those chemicals are removed from their body and they no longer expose themselves to those toxins, the symptoms may reverse. I suffered for years with chronic bronchitis, I observed in myself how exposure to chemicals and this condition went hand and hand.

What is Chemical Intolerance (CI)? Chemical Intolerance is defined as an individual with severe MCS whose symptoms graduate past sensitivity and into "the lack of ability to endure."[1] This means Chemical Intolerance is ***life threatening*** and the individual will longer properly metabolize petroleum based chemicals from any source. With CI the body's biochemical metabolic processes needed to sustain life, are now dysfunctional and at risk for failure. CI compromises the body's biochemical metabolic processes needed to sustain life.

Chemical Intolerance is a recognized medical diagnosis, whereas multiple chemical sensitivity, is not. Multiple Chemical Sensitivity nor MCS is a term not currently recognized by the American Academy of Allergy and Immunology or by the American Medical Association as an established organic disease.

What is Environmental Illness (EI)? Environmental Illness or EI, is defined as an individual whose sensitivity extends beyond the usual allergic reaction to pollen, mold, dust, mites, and chemicals. The EI individual can be sensitive to anything in the environment include, but are not limited to:

- Electricity
- Asbestos
- Lead
- Mercury
- Cadmium
- Fiberglass

As well as environmental energy fields such as electromagnetic and environmental forces, like too much heat or cold. Electromagnetic fields (EMF) include, but are not limited to man-made fields from:

- Atomic radiation
- Base stations
- CERN
- Computers
- Electric motors
- HAARP
- Hair dryers
- Mobile phones
- Power lines
- Radios
- TVs

EI also includes naturally occurring environmental forces such as geopathic stress, extremes in weather, and space energies like neutrino and gamma rays.

What is Idiopathic Environmental Intolerance (IEI)?
Idiopathic Environmental Intolerance or IEI, is an umbrella term which incorporate MCS and EI. The use of IEI as a catchall diagnoses, was too broad. Another term for IEI is Multiple Chemical Sensitivities Syndrome or MCSS. This was a label used by the World Health Organization until the term Idiopathic Environmental Intolerance was introduced as well as the term "Electric hypersensitivity" or EHS.

Therefore, for a few years at least, the current preferred medical term throughout world was Idiopathic Environmental Intolerance, or IEI. The word idiopathic is a medical term that simply means "a disease without apparent or known cause" and in this case the unknown cause is coming from the environment. Environmental factors, chemicals, natural and unnatural forces are too vast, and we just don't need anymore letters and labels!

8

We need solutions.

After thirty plus years of living with this problem I have come to understand this is a modern epidemic. It's a big jigsaw puzzle to piece together and one of the corner pieces is knowing a little bit of history.

It wasn't until 1989 when the first surveys went out to 89 clinicians and researchers with the goal of defining this controversial syndrome known as Multiple Chemical Sensitivity. Ten years later during the first consensus held in 1999 science arrived at six symptoms that define multiple chemical sensitivity. Researchers and clinicians from the United States and Canada,[2] took a great deal of time to narrow down the criteria for MCS, searching through vast and varied theories in order to begin the research for a drug cure.

Research Science's Clinical Criteria for MCS:

1. *"The symptoms are reproducible with [repeated chemical] exposure."*
2. *"The condition is chronic."*
3. *"Low levels of exposure [lower than previously or commonly tolerated] result in manifestations of the syndrome."*
4. *"The symptoms improve or resolve when the incidents are removed."*
5. *"Responses occur to multiple [chemically unrelated] substances."*
6. *"Symptoms involve multiple organs."*

Most of the information you will find online is from the 1999 Consensus Report. I will be taking you up several levels with my information. What you will find in this book took over thirty years of personal experience and observations. A story that ends with a healthy and vibrant pain free individual. What I will be sharing with you goes beyond theories and heads straight into how.

How I overcame, how I survived and now thrive where many have not.[3]

From my thirty years of personal research I have not witnessed any progression of theories into a drug cure or medical treatment for multiple chemical sensitives. In my opinion, this puts research science at the front end of the problem, and the signatories to the Consensus Report given at the National Institutes of Health in 1999 at the Atlanta Conference[4] and the Research and Update Recommendations in 2009-2013 for the Gulf War Veteran[5] agree with me.

When science reduces our symptoms into a defined set of criteria to manage symptoms, then begin an expensive pursuit of a drug cure, this is an example of reductionism[6] in science.

Reductionism

In science, something the average person may not be aware of is the historical use of reductionism. Reductionism is a method of scientific study where the object of study is reduced down to its smallest parts.[7] This approach works brilliantly for understanding and creating cars, satellites, aircraft, and other complicated machines. However, when reductionism is used in the study of living things it leads to the reductionist conclusion 'that to understand the whole one must reduce it down to its smallest parts', leading one to assume that once you understand the parts, you understand the whole. That mindset ultimately fails in the study of living things, specifically humans. Robert Becker, a pioneer researcher in the field of regeneration of living things, clearly found that *"The living human body will always be more than the sum of its parts."*[8]

To date, researchers and doctors have not come to a solution for those with:
- Multiple Chemical Sensitivity (MCS)
- Chemical Intolerance (CI)

- Environmental Illness (EI)
- Idiopathic Environmental Intolerance (IEI)

MCS, CI, EI, and IEI individuals are not being helped by today's status quo of reductionism in science. The fate for those suffering with EI and IEI is all to often labeled as a mental illness. In my experience, after I was diagnosed and properly labeled I was still sick and my only solution from science was to be reduced to live a limited lifestyle of avoidance. This ultimately included what I ate, put on my body and what I inhaled.

We are each an individual and a unique collection of our thoughts, emotions, foods, inner environments, and DNA as well as family history, soul history, soul mission, and physical makeup. Reductionism in science hits the end of its chain with the MCS and EI individual, and these limitations become glaringly obvious as the MCS individual spirals into CI and on into liver failure or the EI individual spirals out of society and away from the painful EMFs. The idea that every single human being should be able to tolerate every single man made chemical and aberrant frequency *indefinitely,* is ludicrous and insulting to the natural world.

Did any of these scientists stop to think that perhaps these people with MCS, CI, EI, and IEI are actually closer to a normal than they realize?

Within these pages I will do my humble best to explain each of these avenues of Tomorrow's Medicine in simple everyday language. With this opening into the truth may your own insights give way to a new paradigm of what real health is and how to achieve it for yourself.

When I share my story, I feel whole and complete. I feel that all the pain and illness I have gone through has not been in vain. Instead I feel inspired that I may give another person hope where there was none. No one has had the same experience that I had.

No one has had the same experience that you've had. Of this, I'm sure, because you're a unique individual complete in your own experiences. I am writing this book to help you on your unique journey into the well-being of homeostasis.

I desire to be the voice of hope and strength, to be a worthy companion to assist you in your own personal journey with Multiple Chemical Sensitivity (MCS), Chemical Intolerance (CI), Environmental Illness (EI), and Idiopathic Environmental Intolerance (IEI).

<u>Chapter One</u>

Experience is Knowledge

"The meaning of the word "truth" varies according to whether we deal with a fact of experience, a mathematical proposition, or a scientific theory."
~Albert Einstein~

It's important for sufferers and their loved ones to understand that the symptoms of Multiple Chemical Sensitivity (MCS), Chemical Intolerance (CI), Environmental Illness (EI) and Idiopathic Environmental Intolerance (IEI) can differ from person to person. The severity of the reaction is also different and unique to the individual. Symptoms can be random, acute and annoying or chronic and life threatening.

The following is a list of possible symptoms based on my personal experience and what others suffering from MCS, CI, EI, and IEI have shared with me. This list may seem excessive, however, understand, the vast and varied possible symptoms are one of medical science's conundrums and why the medical profession has such a difficult time with the diagnosis. (*Please note: This list is alphabetized for your convenience and a space to note your personal symptoms.)

_____Abdominal Cramping
_____Acid Reflux
_____Aching Joints
_____Acne
_____Adult Acne
_____Age and Liver Spots
_____Allergy(s)
_____Alternating Chills, Sweats, Weak, Trembling with Bowel Movement
_____Apathy

14

_____Anger
_____Anxiety
_____Auto Immunity Disorders
_____Acquired Immune Disorders

_____Bad Body Odor
_____Bad Breath, and Bad Taste in Mouth
_____Blisters Without Cause
_____Blood Disorders
_____Blood Sugar Imbalance
_____Bloating
_____Brain Fog
_____Breast Enlargement by Swelling
_____Breathing Difficulties
_____Bronchitis
_____Bone Loss
_____Burning Bladder
_____Burning Sensation Urinating
_____Buzz in Fingertips, Face or Traveling up Arms or Legs

_____Candida Overgrowth
_____Cancer
_____Cellular Diseases, Lysosomal Rupture
_____Clothing in Certain Colors Uncomfortable
_____Confusion
_____Cough
_____Chest Tightness
_____Cholesterol
_____Connective Tissue Dysfunction
_____Constipation
_____Cuticles Spilts, Bleeds

_____DNA Mutations
_____Dental Troubles
_____Dermatitis
_____Defatting Dermatitis
_____Depression
_____Diarrhea

_____Diabetes not Controllable
_____Difficulty in Conceiving, after a Fun Year of Trying
_____Difficulty Passing Urine
_____Digestive Troubles End to End
_____Discomfort In Polyester Clothing
_____Dizziness
_____Dystonia
_____Dry Aging Skin

_____Earaches: Chronic and Acute
_____Erratic Menstrual Cycle
_____Electric Tingles and Shocks in Face, Fingertips, Limbs
_____Emotions
_____Endocrine System-Hypo or Hyper Disorders of:
    _____Pineal
    _____Hypothalamus
    _____Pituitary
    _____Parathyroid
    _____Thyroid
    _____Thymus
    _____Pancreas
    _____Reproductive System
_____Endometriosis
_____Enlarged Prostate
_____Erectile Dysfunction
_____Extreme Ear Wax or Fluid
_____Eyes: Easily Tearing or Burning
_____Eyes: Sensitive to Sunlight

_____Face Tingles with Electrical Buzz
_____Fainting
_____Fatigue
_____Feet Stench
_____Feelings of Being Crazy
_____Fertility Problems
_____Fibromyalgia
_____Foggy Thinking

____Genetic Concerns
____Gum Issues

____Hair: Dull, Oily, Dry
____Hair Loss
____Headaches
____Heart Palpitations
____Hormone Imbalances
____Hypersensitivity
____Hyper Reactions
____Hysteria
____Hypoglycemia

____Immune System Weak
____Impotence
____Impulsive Behavior
____Inability to Lose Weight
____Itchy Eyes
____Incontinence
____Infertility
____Inflammation, Swelling
____Intestines: Overactive, Underachieving, and Leaking
____Insomnia
____Irritability

____Joints, Cartilage, Ligaments: Creaking, Cracking

____Liver Disorders
____Lack of Motivation
____Loss of Interest in Sex
____Lack of Sex Drive
____Laziness
____Leaky Gut
____Leg Muscle Cramps
____Lips Tingling
____Liver Spots
____Liver Issues
____Lowered Immune Response
____Lowered Libido

_____Low Blood Sugar
_____Low Sperm Count
_____Lysosomal Rupture

_____Malaise
_____Memory Loss
_____Mental Confusion
_____Menopause Madness
_____Menopause Symptoms
_____Mental Illness: Anxiety, Depression, Paranoia
_____Migraines
_____Missed Periods with No Conception
_____Mood Swings
_____Muscle Cramps, Distortion
_____Muscles Weakness: Easily Injured

_____Nausea
_____Nails: Deformed Nail Bed
_____Nervous System
_____Nose Pain
_____Nose Swelling
_____Nose: Splitting Interior
_____Night Sweats

_____Obesity
_____Obsessive Thoughts
_____Osteoporosis, Osteopenia
_____Overweight

_____Paranoia
_____Pain: Anywhere and Everywhere
_____Painful Emotions
_____Painful Fingers
_____Painful Feet
_____Painful Jaw
_____Painful Joints
_____Pain on Left Side
_____Painful Mouth
_____Painful Muscles

_____Painful Nerves
_____Painful Nose
_____Pain on Right Side
_____Painful Scalp
_____Painful Skin
_____Painful Toes
_____Panic
_____Personality Changes
_____PMS, PMDD
_____Polyester Clothing Uncomfortable
_____Prostate Cancer
_____Prostate Inflammation

_____Rage
_____Rapid Weight Loss
_____Rapid Weight Gain or Swelling
_____Rashes
_____Red Hot Spots on Joints
_____Red Dots on Skin
_____Reduced Muscular Strength
_____Respiratory Stress
_____Reproductive Issues
_____Runny Nose
_____Runny Ears
_____Runny Eyes

_____Sensitivities
_____Sensitive Skin
_____Sinus Headaches
_____Sinus: Irritated
_____Scalp Pain
_____Spleen Troubles
_____Skeletal Weakness
_____Skin Splits or Separates into Lines
_____Skipped or Missed Periods without Conception
_____Sleepiness
_____Slow Recovery from Surgery
_____Scratchy Throat
_____Sore Throat

_____Sudden Loss of Consciousness
_____Sudden Runny Nose
_____Sudden Weakness
_____Swollen Areas on Inner Lips of Vulva
_____Swollen Feet / Ankles
_____Swollen Organs

_____Trembling on Toilet During Bowel Movements
_____Thyroid Symptoms, Hyper or Hypo
_____Thoughts of Suicide or Impending Death
_____Tooth and Bone Loss

_____Urinary System Disorders
_____Underweight
_____Uncontrollable Crying
_____Upset Stomach

_____Vertigo

_____Water Retention
_____Weakness
_____Weeping With Excessive Emotions
_____Weeping Fluid from Skin

You may be thinking, with so many symptoms, how do I know if these are actually related to:

- Multiple Chemical Sensitivity (MCS)
- Chemical Intolerance (CI)
- Environmental Illness (EI)
- Idiopathic Environmental Intolerance (IEI)

Good question. Let's take it one step further by asking yourself these next questions. If you find yourself relating to any of the following scenarios, it's highly likely that you may be suffering from MCS, CI, EI, and IEI.

When you walk into the laundry detergent aisle at the grocery store does your nose run? Does the detergent aisle give you a headache or leave you feeling sick and/or tired? Does pumping gas make you feel ill? Do the perfume displays make you nauseous? Do you feel sick in environments with fresh paint, cleaning supplies, or plug-in type air fresheners?

Do you get sick easily and suddenly? Are headaches, sore throats, and sinus infections a part of your everyday life? Is your skin sensitive, tender, red, rough, cracking, splitting, excessively dry, or oily? Do you have a rash for no reason? Have you ever had an unexplained rash appear after wearing dry cleaned or new clothing? Have you become suddenly exhausted trying on new clothing? Do some fabrics and fabric colors bother you? Do people think you are eccentric because you dislike certain fabrics or colors? Is dermatitis ruining your love life? Do you even feel like having a love life?

Do you avoid hugging certain people because they wear cologne? Does your nose suddenly start running for no obvious reason? Do you feel shooting pains or random electrical tingling sensations in your body? Do your eyes burn or does your nose run when someone new walks into the room? Does your nose run or face buzz when you walk into a new environment? Have you ever felt lightheaded or felt your lips tingle when walking into a new environment? Has your chest ever tightened and/or your breathing become labored for no apparent reason? Do you suddenly become overwhelmed by anxiety without an obvious cause?

Have you ever eaten food that put you into a coughing spasm or a sneezing fit? Have you eaten food that just would not digest or gave you acid reflux? Is inflammation anywhere in your body a problem? Do you have inflammation in your digestive system? Do you suspect you have leaky gut?

Do you get the flu or flu like symptoms that just will not go away? Do you have severe symptoms that overwhelm you and then nothing happens for a long period of time? Do you have symptoms such as lingering fatigue and a general sense of the blahs? Do you lack ambition and motivation? As a result of these feelings are you accused of being lazy, a hypochondriac or an oddball?

Do you swell in certain areas of your body? Are you overweight with a distorted abdomen and tapering arms and legs? Are your upper arms and thighs oversized and swollen? Are you accused of overeating?

Sometimes the suffering goes unnoticed by others because you don't look sick in the typical way that most people expect. There are no fevers or gushing blood to prove that you are feeling awful and that your energy is draining away.

These scenarios have been reported by myself and others suffering with:

- Multiple Chemical Sensitivity (MCS)
- Chemical Intolerance (CI)
- Environmental Illness (EI)
- Idiopathic Environmental Intolerance (IEI)

Relating to the above situations is a huge clue that you too could be a chemically/environmentally sensitive individual.

I was once bombarded with these symptoms, and eventually overwhelmed by them. I noticed, as I recovered with the solutions I will discuss throughout the book, many of the symptoms that once were persistent annoyances, have left my life. Some symptoms are completely gone and others have been reduced to the point that they no longer interfere with the quality of my life, or with my ability to go places and do the things I need or want to do.

We're all assaulted daily with numerous chemicals and they're coming at us in every direction. They are in the air. They are in the water. They are in our body products. They are in our clothes. They are in our food. They are in the land. They are in our medicine. They are everywhere.

Your body is not betraying you. In these pages, I will share with you who your true betrayers are. Your body is trying to get your attention with all that pain. In a way, pain is your friend. It's an alarm system sounding off, "Alert! Alert! Something's not right here!" Ignoring pain and discomfort or changes in your body, or masking it with medications will never address the true underlying issues that your body is begging you to address.

My encounters with chemical sensitivities began in 1981. I have noticed the same symptoms in my children and grandchildren. I have also noticed these same indicators in people around me, and even pets.

For me, it took lots of money, courage, and time before I received the medical diagnosis of Chemical Intolerance. Back then staying alive became the focus in everything I did. Today my focus is to share everything I've learned or discovered about chemicals and the environment and their effects on the human body as well as what solutions worked for me as I dealt with:

- Multiple Chemical Sensitivity (MCS)
- Chemical Intolerance (CI)
- Environmental Illness (EI)
- Idiopathic Environmental Intolerance (IEI)

I fooled myself into thinking I was safe from chemicals because I followed my doctor's orders such as avoiding items containing the offending chemicals. I was totally unaware of the impending danger I was in. For me there were serious consequences to being exposed to various chemicals and substances found in everyday life. You or your loved ones may also have severe reactions to everyday chemicals. It's important to note that these chemicals can have a far greater effect on your children, grandchildren and pets.

Although I had extensive medical tests supporting the seriousness of my medical condition, my health care providers could offer little to help me. My diagnosis had little value because the only solution the doctors could offer was chemical avoidance. That's proved impossible chemicals are everywhere! It took me years to find the solutions that I'm now sharing with you in this book; solutions that although safe and effective, are not not main stream knowledge.

Doctors don't have the time to search in earnest as I had to do. Researchers as I mentioned earlier are using the scientific method of reductionism to seek answers and understand the problem by reducing the body down to its parts as if it were a car. I'm going to share with you why this reductionistic approach is not working for the chemical/environmental sensitive individual. In my opinion, the reductionist approach is missing the problem, which reduces people like us to staying home, reducing our choices, and reducing our life span. There is another way, another route that I took and it has made all the difference to my life, and perhaps it can for you as well.

My diagnosis confused my family, friends, employers, and my co-workers. They were also invested in the established belief system regarding health and most of them couldn't understand why there was no "pill" for me. Therefore over the decades I have frequently encountered impatience. I needed more than to simply avoid chemicals. That's impossible! Chemicals are everywhere!

I was determined to find a solution.

First, I had to make a plan. That started with investigating what I could and could not tolerate. I needed to know what would be acceptable to stay healthy and alive and what would not. I applied this idea to all areas of my life. Everything was under scrutiny: food, the environment, my current knowledge, information presented to me as well as career choices. I had to leave people and circumstances behind that would not respect what I needed in my life. I needed to stay well at all costs.

I saved my life, on my own, at home.

I did not accept the finality of fact that there were no answers from the western medical model. I did not lose faith when the eastern medicine model told me the chemical burden was too great. I rejected the prognosis of both cultures and turned within, surrendering to my intuition. In doing so, I discovered a new way of dealing with the multitude of chemical challenges ... a way that worked!

I have put together the keys to the solution and it's more than avoidance or accepting the status quo. It's an actual solution. Under the definition of the word **cure:**[1] *"recovery or relief from a disease."* I believe I have indeed found something better than "a cure" for the **dis-ease** of a body fighting for it's life in a world awash with chemicals. However, since I'm not offering you a drug and I'm not a doctor, I cannot offer you a "cure"[2] as it's against the law in most parts of the United States. According to the regulations of many state laws, only drugs and medical procedures using drugs are what cure (anything else is happenstance). The FDA has firm perimeters around who and what can cure and treat.[3]

I have been researching this subject for many years and when I found my solutions the search was over. When I had my epiphany and began to compile my information to write this book I was rather surprised. After all these years of searching for answers in libraries, that in today's world of technology, sparse new information was available and no solutions were being offered by main stream science. I was annoyed with finding the same limited thinking I ran into decades ago. Main stream science is no closer to a cure or treatment in 2015 than they were in 1981!

Another observation I made on the subject of Multiple Chemical Sensitivity (MCS), Chemical Intolerance (CI), Environmental Illness (EI), and Idiopathic Environmental Intolerance (IEI) was the same old stigma of, *it's all in your head.*[4] This has been a response for other ailments that had been dismissed in the past, but are finally now recognized as real, such as Fibromyalgia and PMS. Even today as I finish this book in 2015, I find the same old information[5] and new theories with a pretty odd names like, Orthorexia nervosa[6] and Methylenetetrahydrofolate Reductase (MTHFR).[7] Research slants this in a way that places all the blame of our sickness on our genes. I find their observations unsettling and misdirected, leading us to a false belief that our gift of sensitivities are some how a flaw. A subconscious belief in a flaw can do tremendous damage to the body, as Bruce Lipton, the world renowned cell biologist, and self proclaimed spiritual scientist laid out for us in *The Biology of Belief.*

Therefore in order to share with you fully and completely how I survived, I must share an intimate layer of myself; my spiritual knowing. It's the base of what got me this far and is a very important aspect of my healing journey. I understand that we all have our own beliefs. It's not my intention to alienate anyone, so I just want to warn you ahead of time that I will be using terms like God and Universe and other spiritual terms like Angels and Ascended Masters, feel free to replace these ideas and terms with your own spiritual beliefs.

We are a divine creative spirit within a body, here in this dimension to manifest reality in our own unique way. As I became aware of my inner connection with the divine, creative, loving, energy of the Universe I came to understand I was a reflection of this energy and here to be a creator of my own reality via my thoughts, actions, and feelings. This can be hard to do when you aren't feeling well.

One can stay alive for some time without entertaining God's divine energy, but if one wants to **thrive** with these conditions then a new paradigm must be explored. Not one bit of research I found in the years before I found my solutions addressed the spiritual side of these troubling conditions. Anyone this far in their search for relief deserves to know the whole truth.

God does not make junk.

My grandmother had a little shop with a sign over her cash register that said, "I know I'm special because God does not make junk." Could we all just step back, take a deep breath, and think about that?

God gave you a beautiful work of art, the human body. The human body is designed with systems created to protect you from impending danger. That body will respond to your every command. Treat it well and pay attention. Your body communicates beautifully with you. You on the other hand may not be listening. When you and your body are communicating with affinity for the environment, this shared reality becomes the state of homeostasis.[8]

Homeostasis: is when the body is in perfect balance. When the body is in perfect balance, it's ability to respond and adjust to disruptive changes is increased. The highest achievement you can do for your body is to attain and remain in homeostasis.

Would you like to be a better communicator with your body? Would you feel better if you knew you were actually doing the things your body needs and wants. Instead, are you struggling each day to get out of bed? Do you feel you are sliding backwards into disease, instead of moving forward into homeostasis?

The process of how I came to understand what my body was saying to me came slowly through the years. With each search and discovery of a real solution I would increase my immune response. One day I finally "got it," I heard the message of my body, I listened and eventually I began moving forward into homeostasis. I became well.

Searching with hope is how I conquered crippling chemical intolerance and now live easier with my sensitivities and allergies. This is also how you may be able to live with a healthier body in a toxic world.

I DID IT
and if I can do it that means it's possible...

YOU COULD TOO!

There is hope.

<u>Chapter Two</u>

Looking for a Cure in All the Wrong Places

"Perfection of means and confusion of goals seem, in my opinion, to characterize our age."
~Albert Einstein~

Not so long ago medicine was made from plants. Today pharmaceutical drugs are **synthetic** versions of medicinal plants created in a lab **from man-made chemicals** instead of plants. The reason for this? **Mother Earth's plants cannot be patented.**

Mother Nature created plants to nurture all humans and animals, *the earthlings.* Fewer and fewer of us know the healing power of nature. Drug companies, bio-tech industries, and food manufacturers don't make the big bucks from plants. The biggest profits come from patented synthetic versions of plants used in drugs,[1] cosmetics and other consumer products.

On June 30, 1906 Congress passed the first Food and Drug Act and the first food and drug lobbyist was born. These are the *Agents Provocateur* aka *Lobbyists* for corporations such as pharmaceutical, bio-tech, food and cosmetic manufacturers and suppliers to these industries. This is just to give you an idea of who has the massive financial resources to purchase, oops, I mean persuade enough change to relax laws, sidestep enforcement of procedures, ignore conflicting research, and control the information on labeling. The lobbyist are always busy in Washington and not many of them are working for our best interests. As an example, currently some of these companies are spending millions to hide the truth from the public through individual State Food Labeling initiatives, as well as federal regulations.

Drug companies pay extraordinary amounts of money for third party public relations firms to create publicity campaigns designed to give you warm fuzzy feelings with a finely crafted message that "all is well" when you take this pill, suppress a symptom or smear something somewhere on your body. Then the images on the screen often don't match the list of side effects delivered in a low tone, fast talking dismissive voice. This is how the Profiteers run their game on you, and walk away with minor fines compared to their massive profits.[2]

Examples of lobbyists and marketing succeeding during the 20th century include the 1958 Federal Food Additive Amendment, which relaxed the enforcement of the 1938 Federal Food, Drug and Cosmetics Act. This amendment to the 1938 Food and Drug Act, tainted the American food supply for the multiple chemically sensitive individual. It exempted food additives placed on the "Generally Regarded As Safe" (GRAS) and allowed these food additives to remain on the GRAS list without updated testing. The Delaney Clause added to the 1958 Amendment, is a provision within the amendment clearly stating that any chemical additive found to induce cancer in man or after animal testing, is found to induce cancer in animals cannot be added to our food. This law is being ignored, skirted and broken in spirit and word.

In 1962 the Kefauver-Harris Amendment placed the responsibility for proving the safety and efficiency of the drug with the manufacturer,[3] and thereby loosening enforcement of testing procedures used for products placed on the Generally Regarded As Safe (GRAS) list.[4]

This practice continues, allowing the safety and efficiency testing to be conducted by the very pharmaceutical companies that make the drugs. It's common for the process of proving a drug's safety and efficiency to take a shorter time frame than it does to remove a drug from the marketplace once it has proven to have harmful side effects. This process of drug safety being handled in-house is not a good idea in my opinion.

I don't know about your house, but at my house it would be like leaving a three-year old in charge of the refrigerator. Things are going to be messy, missing, and sticky. There will be no acceptance of responsibility from the three-year old! She will blame everything on the refrigerator, just like the scientific community blames your response to chemical sensitivity on your body! Instead of placing the responsibility on the food and drugs you ingest, which are made synthetically with chemicals.

As I said earlier, there was a time when medicine was made from plants. Today very few drugs are made from actual plants, instead pharmaceutical drugs are patented synthetic versions of medicinal plants created in a lab from man-made chemicals. There are a few new pharmaceutical drugs (called Biologics and Biosimilars) derived from live animal cell proteins, unfortunately these drug and are wildly expensive to develop, and not likely suitable for chemical sensitive people as these proteins require chemicals for stabilization.[5]

Even today when searching for plant based medicine you will find that most plant based drugs are actually just simple synthetic modifications or copies of the naturally obtained phytochemical substances. Phytochemical is the naturally occurring chemical within a plant.[6] Today there very few drugs that are simple phytochemical drugs.

The majority of pharmaceutical drugs made today originate from the following three sources:[7]

- Bacteria/Mold/Fungus Extracts
- Benzene Derivative
- Chlorine

These three poisons are the basic building blocks of modern pharmaceutical medicine. My research and experience show they're also the primary antagonists responsible for creating sensitivity within the human body. This, I believe, is why people with chemical/environmental sensitivity will never find a cure in a drug. Some believe that manmade benzene/chlorine/mold based chemical compounds are not a problem. I strongly disagree. I'm not able to reside in the same environment with any of these three, much less have them injected into or ingested by my body.

The Solution is Easier Than Finding a Cure

How can anyone with chemical sensitivities resolve their problem with more chemicals? How are you going to get well with a drug whose molecular base component is benzene or chlorine, the very chemicals that caused the sensitivity?

Benzene is on the Center for Disease Control's known carcinogen list.[8]

Chlorine is one of the most toxic and reactive elements for humans.[9] Researchers around the world and in the United States have found that water disinfected with chlorine can react with organic material and create a type of chemical compound called trihalomethanes.[10] (sounds like: try hall o meth anes). Trihalomethanes or THM can be inhaled, ingested, and then accumulated in the fat cells. Some herbicides, fungicides, and insecticides are manufactured using chlorine attached to a carbon molecule thus creating a synthetic structure that becomes trapped in the human fat cells after inhalation and or ingestion. Researcher's findings in Norway[11] and New Zealand[12] support that chlorine disinfection of water creates byproducts that can cause cancer, birth defects, and spontaneous miscarriages!

I assure you, if you are a chemical/environmental sensitive; mold, chlorine or benzene based drugs are not going to be a drug that positively changes your life for you. It's going to require returning to some very simple ideas.

You can bake a cake out of flour or you can bake a cake out of something that looks like flour, something like talc powder.[13] Do you want a cake of talc powder or flour? We can clearly see the absurdity of consuming fake food, *why don't we see the absurdity of synthetic medicine?* Synthetic food additives, benzene and chlorine based medications aren't the best option for people with Multiple Chemical Sensitivities (MCS), or Chemical Intolerance (CI).

Let's get back to basics.

1. Get your mind off drugs, out of the hospital, and out into the fresh air.
2. Get back to where you came from - **nature**. You are a product of nature not a product of the hospital, *so stop* looking there for answers they do *not* have.

The hospital is for trauma. The hospital understands broken pieces and how to put them back together again. The hospital built by pharmacopoeia does not fully understand the chemically intolerant/environmentally sensitive individual.

To those who feel that manmade benzene based chemicals compounds are not the problem, I encourage you to read on. In the following chapters I will do my best to explain how and why these chemicals are so dangerous. My goal is to help you understand why drugs made from benzene and chlorine chemicals are not a solution for chemically sensitive people. You will see that these ingredients are one of the "mysteries" killing us as a species by creating a multitude of problems such as:

- Brain Damage
- Cancer
- Infertility
- Nerve Damage
- Organs: Swollen or Shrinking
- Premature Aging and Death

Those of you that were pinning your hopes on a drug cure may be feeling a little bit of despair right now. Please don't!!!

Instead, know that you don't need to continue to aggravate your chemical sensitivities past your physical and emotional tolerance.

Thankfully, there are **Alternate Solutions.**

PART TWO:

The Experience

To understand where I'm coming from you have to understand a little of who I am, where I've been, and what I've experienced. You may find bits and pieces of yourself within my personal story.

<u>Chapter Three</u>

How Does Someone Get Like This?

*"In order to be an immaculate member of a flock of sheep,
one must above all be a sheep oneself."*
~Albert Einstein~

My earliest memories are of army bases, moving boxes, my mom unpacking them, and my dad telling me little moron jokes. Some of the wisdom I found to be most profound, may be steeped in little moron stories.

"What did the little moron say when he was caught digging through all the horse manure?" my Dad would ask.

"What?" I would ask.

"With all this horse manure, there must be a pony in here somewhere!" My Dad with his Texan accent would answer with his affected little moron voice.

To my preschooler sense of humor that silly voice was the highlight of the joke.

From those early formative years I would learn that everything is temporary and it's best to laugh at the ridiculousness of it all. This would prove to be an invaluable tool for the survival of my mental health as I ran the chemical gauntlet during my young adulthood.

I remember being five and telling my grandfather, Papa that the food tasted strange. The chicken smelled funny and the tomatoes had no flavor at all. I clearly remember him saying to me, "that's because that is store bought food."

I didn't understand and must have looked puzzled because

he continued with "By the time you grow up and are my age (he was probably 50 at the time) the food will not be worth eating." He was right.

That conversation comes back to me frequently, especially as I slosh through the chemical laden food offerings fifty years later. On that day, long ago I revealed that I knew the difference. Through taste I knew if we were eating store bought food or food from my Great Grandmother Bessie's lakeside garden or my Papa's city garden. Smell could tell me if the chicken was store bought or one of Grandma Bessie's free roaming, bug and worm-eating hens. This time in my life marks the beginning of my development as a sensory food detective and culinary eccentric.

In my childhood I grew up with parents that did not stop the pursuit of knowledge, for themselves, or for their children. Both of my parents sought and completed higher educational degrees in between kids, war, parties, and moving. My father has a fascination for the unexplainable, things like UFOs, politics, and Atlantis. My childhood home was full of books, newspapers, and magazines. Of all the information available in my environment, I found the subjects of UFOs and Atlantis most interesting.

My parents were the best, especially for a kid like me. To develop into a critical thinker I needed to have a free range brain, roaming through any book I found interesting. In my childhood trips to the library were at the top of my fun list. Learning with an open mind and humor is what got me through the experiences I've had with my health.

As a kid, I'd have unexplained rashes. No matter what it looked like, I was told it was prickly heat. Although, sometimes the rashes would appear when it wasn't summer. On two occasions I fainted while having my hair done. As an adult I would learn (from reading Material Safety Data Sheets and government publications) that sudden loss of consciousness or fainting is a symptom of benzene exposure. Many hair products are full of benzene based solvents. Go grab any shampoo bottle and see for yourself.

Sudden sore throats were another symptom of exposure that I would experience. Now I know this was my immune response weakened by environmental chemicals and being overtaken by opportunistic infections. On several occasions I threw up immediately after eating. No one else would get sick. I would just vomit without warning. Later I would connect that reaction with eating food processed with chemical laden oils, flavorings, and preservatives.

By the time I was a teenager, the beginnings of chemical sensitivity were evident, but still we didn't connect the dots. My younger brother had extreme and life threatening allergies. My mother was often overwhelmed by his needs, and so my odd symptoms that occurred early in life, often went unnoticed. We're trained by society to have the attitude: "Oh, that's nothing, insignificant". However, small warnings are very often an indication of a very large "iceberg" hidden beneath the surface.

At the beginning of the tenth grade, all the skin on the inside of my lower lip peeled peeled away (one of the tips of the iceberg). Each day it got worse until skin was peeling off the outside of my lower lip and down onto my chin, leaving a raw area. I remember getting better after spending a few days at home. When I returned to school and consumed an orange flavored drink it instantly created a problem with my lip again. The correlation between food and it's influence on my body began to emerge... right smack on my face.

All through my teen years and into college I had an occasional painful menstrual period often accompanied by, oddly enough, either a sore throat or a bad headache. In college, I had migraine headaches from my periods that put me in bed for a day or two (tips of the icebergs being ignored). The older I got the longer it took to recover from the migraines.

One month such a period I was having! Complete with a bad headache, cramps and feeling sick to my stomach. I took two Midols® for pain. My next memory is waking up in the emergency room. I had passed out from the medication! That was a big clue that something was not right. I left the hospital with a diagnosis of *allergy to aspirin.*

The episode with the Midol® took place in 1973. During my research years later I stumbled upon a big clue. Until about 1972 aspirin had been made from the plant bark of the white willow tree. By 1974 all aspirin was made from the benzene based substitute instead of actual white willow bark.

As I mentioned earlier, pharmaceutical companies are able to copy plants and make synthetic versions of the real plant using the benzene molecule as the base ingredient. This synthetic version made from the benzene molecule now qualifies for a patent. This explains why we have so many benzene based medicines today. Our bodies' reactions to benzene, however, are an indication that this methodology is flawed, and very wrong. We need to get back to nature.

<u>Chapter Four</u>

Trusting Nature

"Look into nature,
and then you will understand it better."
~Albert Einstein~

The first time I remember listening to my inner self and standing up against the status quo of the medical environment was in my early twenties. As I entered into adulthood I was having a happy life. I had graduated from college, started my career, married, and two years into marriage I was having my first baby.

We were so excited, but I was underweight by fifteen pounds at the end of my first trimester. My doctor instructed me to give up salt, spinach, turnip greens, kale, and cabbage; along with several other favorite fruits and vegetables. Instead, I was given a list of foods allowing fast food burgers, steak, and lots of milk and cheese. I was to eat three full meals a day and two snacks. Obediently I complied. By the time I delivered my baby I had gained 65 pounds over my pre-pregnancy weight. My perfect baby girl weighed in as a petite, healthy seven pounder.

My conflicts started soon after delivery. The nursing staff became concerned because I had a very bad headache. My doctor was prescribing Tylenol® for the headache as it was non-aspirin and very "safe." The nurse assured me I wouldn't have an allergic reaction to it, however, I found that the Tylenol® seemed to make the headache worse and I also became very irritable.

When I refused to take the Tylenol® on the next round of drug pushing, the head nurse said that I couldn't go home if I had a headache. She suggested that I take the Tylenol®, even if it was not helping. Her ridiculous logic increased the throbbing in my head. The next day the doctor's orders were to drink three bottles of apple juice and a pitcher of water, and thankfully, no mention of Tylenol®.

Poof! The headache vanished. I had dealt with four highly specialized gynecologists, but the common sense solution came from the eldest doctor on the team. He was a Cuban immigrant whose original medical training came from outside the United States. In Cuba they take a more natural approach to health care.

The hospital staff considered me peculiar because I repeatedly refused to follow maternity ward traditions. One such tradition was the cocktail of injections that automatically came with my hospital room. I refused all the injections for drying up the milk. Instead I continued to fumble through breastfeeding, immune to the disapproving looks and ignoring the formula suggestions. Although I had never actually seen anyone breastfeed a baby, I assured them I was quite capable since I had read several books on the subject. Because of my motherly intuition, I felt sure God would not create babies without providing a perfect food source; all of nature was born with a food source. My inner self knew that perfect food source should be my breasts delivering nourishment to my precious little baby. I stood my ground.

The head nurse was not convinced and didn't understand my reasoning any more than I did hers. To help convince me, or maybe coerce me, they assigned the only male nurse in the maternity ward to care for me. He took his job very seriously and most studiously. That first morning he came in explaining that my breasts must be massaged, lest they become infected. This massage consisted of a rough mauling and rubbing of my round full left breast. I cried with pain and refused to subject the right breast to his educated protocol.

The next day a nurse's aide from one of the Caribbean islands was sent to help me with my nursing. This woman was gentle and experienced. With her kind words and patience it only took a few times and the baby latched on, and contentedly nursed! All was good in my world. A second testament to the value of natural health practices.

A third issue happened later that first day. My hospital roommate's rude husband came in with a cantankerous tone and ended their conversation by lighting up a cigarette in our shared room.

When I requested he put out the cigarette he said in his gravely, macho smoker's voice,

"Why? There are no babies in here," and continued to smoke.

I called the nurse who told him he shouldn't smoke in the room. However, she did not require him to put out the cigarette, and he continued to smoke. He finally put the butt out in his wife's water glass. The year was 1980 and society was deep asleep regarding the dangers of cigarette smoking and especially second hand smoke and its contribution to environmental toxins.

Our bodies have innate intelligence and know how to function. Our bodies know when to begin periods, how and when to deliver babies, how to keep our hearts pumping, and how to operate all the various organs. The maternity ward staff in this situation didn't want to hear what my body was telling me. They didn't trust nature as I did.

This story is critical because it's when I began to trust myself and commit to my decision to trust nature and the body God created. Having a baby changed everything for me. Not only did it make me fully grow up, it helped me become the kind of adult I wanted to be around. It was the first time I had been assertive and stood up for myself and my health. Honoring my intuition and my inner guidance felt different after that experience. I was an adult. I was a mother lion bear goddess as I held my beautiful baby daughter I promised her that I would always do my best to keep us both healthy and safe.

<u>Chapter Five</u>

The Earnest Endocrinologist

"We have to do the best we are capable of. This is our sacred human responsibility."
~Albert Einstein~

At 25 years old, when my baby was about five months old, I had my first post-pregnancy period. It was the worst period of my life. Each month, two weeks before each period, I became an emotional and physical wreck and was absolutely sure I was in hell. I would have either gut-wrenching constipation or life-altering diarrhea. My weight could fluctuate by 15 pounds in just a few days. My mood swings were over the top! All I could do was cry with despair or scream in rage.

As most women do when they have problems associated with their periods, I went to my gynecologist. During the exam my gynecologist performed the standard gynecological exam, listened patiently to my woes, and quickly wrote referrals for two specialist.

The first referral was to an Internist, and the second was for the area's top Endocrinologist. My appointment with the Internist went quickly as we had only a five minute conversation; they drew no blood and took no samples. He quickly dismissed me, referring me on to a Psychiatrist. It took me longer to write my check.

Side Note: Referrals for psychological evaluation are a form of misdiagnosis, a recurring problem for those with MCS, EI, and IEI. Thirty three years later and there's still a misbelief among doctors that their patients are showing signs of anxiety. This is a big controversy in diagnosing MCS, EI, and IEI. Anxiety is not the problem, <u>it's a side effect</u>. Imagine if you had sudden weakness or shortness of breath without explanation, would you not feel anxiety?¹ The question should be asked: *Why* is there anxiety?

The Diagnosis

The second referral was for the area's top endocrinologist. My health insurance did not cover this and he was very expensive. We were blessed when my mother-in-law Muriel, insisted on helping to pay for the additional out-of- pocket expenses.

The phlebotomist took many vials of blood, spent a few hours running a weird machine back and forth over my neck, which intuitively felt wrong. Then I had to pay a big fat bill! I was exhausted. The results of these numerous medical exams determined that I was normal. The science of the day declared me within normal ranges.

The endocrinologist called me back a few weeks later to see if I had improved. I hadn't. I was worse. They drew more blood and subjected me to more lab tests. He was determined to find out why a perfectly healthy woman would be going insane two weeks out of every month. God bless that doctor, he saw his patients as individuals and applied critical thinking to his analysis.

It was a long three-month wait before a nurse from the endocrinologist's office called to schedule a follow up appointment. This was my first doctor consultation that didn't take place in an exam room. I had never actually been inside of a doctor's real office before. The room was full of diplomas, large expensive furniture, and beautiful art. Sitting there among the beauty, the environment made me feel as if I mattered. On that day I felt cared for.

The doctor explained that for some reason the signals in my brain were not responding to pain correctly. At the time, he had no recommendations as it was a new disease. I just remember him using these two new words: "prostaglandin" and "inflammation." He also explained that the symptoms intensified starting with ovulation and continued to strengthen and increase up through the start of menstruation. There was no cure and the researchers were calling it "Pre-menstrual Syndrome" or PMS.

Finally, the crazy periods now had a diagnosis! Yes, I had one of the first medical diagnoses from an endocrinologist for the term Pre-Menstrual Syndrome.[2] No one had heard of PMS except for that earnest endocrinologist and me, until two women that year used PMS as a murder defense in England gaining reduced sentences.[3] PMS now had three ugly sides, two weeks of torment, the potential to deny women high level jobs and custody of their children.[4]

I'm Allergic to What?

In the course of all the previous medical testing revealing the new disease of PMS, the endocrinologist also ran a series of allergy tests. He seemed resigned with me as he delivered the news of the results of the allergy tests. The end results: *a diagnosis for the antigen for toluene.*

"What does that mean?" I asked.

"You're allergic to Toluene." He said matter of fact.

I remember asking him, "What's toluene?"

He responded, "It's the T in BHT."[5]

I was completely baffled by that answer. What were these mystery letters? What did this mean for me? He had a look on his face that told me he didn't know what that meant for me either.

I asked about a prescription for medicine to treat the allergy. I was very disappointed to learn that there was nothing for me to take. He told me to avoid everything with BHT in it. The only recourse was avoiding toluene completely. At that moment I didn't realize the magnitude of this diagnosis. I was about to learn that meant just about everything.

__Chapter Six__

The Mother Solvent

"I believe that the present fashion of applying the axioms of physical science to human life is not only entirely a mistake but has also something reprehensible about it."
~Albert Einstein~

A trip to the library enlightened me to the disturbing fact that toluene was a solvent.[1] A solvent used everyday in pharmaceuticals, chemicals, rubber, and plastics industries. I would also learn that toluene was in detergents but not soaps. The laundry soap I used for the baby's clothes was the only laundry product that didn't have BHT on the label and was a soap. I washed my clothes and her clothes in the laundry soap without BHT and my husband's clothes in a commercial laundry detergent with BHT. Eventually I was washing all sheets and towels with the baby's laundry soap.

That was just the beginning. I next examined the labels on all the beauty products decorating my bathroom windowsill. Following the advice of the endocrinologist, I threw everything out with BHT on the ingredient label. Eventually I felt I had gotten a handle on the BHT.

I was naive. After tossing out everything containing BHT, I would *still* have chemical reactions. It turns out I still had many beauty products made from ingredients with long scientific names that I didn't understand. There were initials *other than* BHT on these labels. I matched up all of the initials with the words from my library research. It took me a few minutes but I began to realize that everything in my shower had toluene *disguised* on the label.

Frustrated and determined to find answers I took several trips to the library. Remember, in 1981, Google was a baby's word and the internet was decades away. As I dug deeper for information at the library I began to understand more and more about the chemicals and initials that were surrounding my life.

I managed to piece together what toluene actually was. Toluene is found naturally in crude oil, forest fires, and the tolu tree, a type of pine tree.[2] Toluene is the base of almost all solvents, (turpentine was the other solvent of the day) and is used in numerous products such as food additives, cosmetics, medicine and engine degreasers. These alternative ingredients include: methyl-benzene", "benzene, methyl", "toluolo", "methacide", and "phenylmethane." I was beginning to see how if one is allergic to toluene one could be allergic to other ingredients with different names in items used on a daily basis.

The definition of toluene[3] is: "*Toluene is a solvent and is also used in organic synthesis, as **a starting material** for the synthesis of _many compounds_,*" Most important for you to understand is those "*_many compounds_*" are what you may unwittingly be eating and using in body care products, medicines and other everyday consumer products.

So how does the natural toluene from crude oil, forest fires and tolu trees become ingredients in this vast array of products? I learned that in petroleum distillation, is:

- The first step is to boil the crude oil.[4]

- The second step is to maximize the capture of the resulting derivatives.[5]

- Benzene and toluene are the first of these derivatives captured, they're also referred to as virgin light and heavy naphtha.[6] [7]

- Toluene and benzene are at the foundation of any given petrochemical product.

- Medicine, vitamins, food additives, solvents, hair dye, nail polish, cosmetics, fragrances, plastics, detergents and more are made from benzene and toluene.[8]

- Today's refining processes now make it possible to extract benzene and toluene from fracking shale.

Facts About Toluene[9]

- Toluene is a clear, toxic, flammable liquid.

- Toluene vapor/air mixtures are explosive.[10]

- Toluene Carries a Health Hazard of 2 (Slightly Hazardous).

- Toluene is used in making fingernail polish, lacquers, paints, paint thinners and rubber, printing, and leather processes.

- Toluene has been detected in maternal milk in human. Passes through the placental barrier in human. Embrotoxic (toxic to embryo) and /or fetotoxic (toxic to fetus) in animal. May cause adverse reproductive effects and birth defects (teratogenic). May affect genetic material (mutagenic).

- IARC (International Agency for Research on Cancer) and the NTP (U.S Department of Toxicology Program) have not listed toluene as a carcinogenic, however as of 2014 the National Toxicology Program reports have labeled toluene as suspected to be a human carcinogen.[11]

- NIOSH (National Institute for Occupational Safety and Health) gives toluene a danger to life or health at a concentration of 500 parts per million.[12]

- Examples of 1 part per million:
    - Four drop of toluene into a 55 gallon drum of water would produce a toluene concentration of 1 part per million.[13]
    - Two thousand drops in that 55 gallons would be equal to a toluene concentration of 500 parts per

        million and a danger to your health.

- One part per million is equal to one penny in ten thousand dollars, therefore if toluene were money, five dollars out of ten thousand dollars would be a danger to your health.

- ATSDR (Agency for Toxic Substance and Disease Registry) gives a minimal inhalation risk of 1 parts per million for acute (short term exposure) and .08 parts per million for chronic (long term exposure).[14]

- OSHA (Occupational Safety & Health Administration) gives fatal concentration estimated to be 1800 to 2000 parts per million for an hour.[15]

- EPA (Environmental Protection Agency) says a person can:
  - Smell toluene in the air at a concentration of 8 parts of toluene per million of air.
  - Taste it in water at a concentration of between 0.04 and 1 parts per million. In our previous example of parts per million, instead of four drops, that would be only one drop of toluene into that 55 gallon drum of water and you would taste the toluene.

- EPA has toluene listed as a hazard waste material and requires proper disposal in a hazard waste site landfill.

- EPA issued a pre-publication in January 2015 announcing that a significant usage change is imminent.[16]

- EPA has concluded that there is inadequate information to assess the carcinogenic potential of toluene. However, you should know what they did find!
  - The EPA has found the highest concentrations of toluene occur in indoor air from the usage of common household products such as:
    - Paint
    - Paint thinners
    - Adhesives

- Synthetic fragrances (such as air fresheners and plug ins)
- Nail polish
- The EPA when measuring toluene in the air using micro grams per cubic meter found levels of toluene in:
    - 1.3 in Rural air
    - 10.8 in Urban air
    - 31.5 Indoor air averaged!

The definition of Benzene[17] is: a liquid chemical that is a colorless volatile toxic liquid aromatic hydrocarbon H_6C_6 *used in organic synthesis...* used to make plastics, fuel for automobiles and other substances.

Facts About Benzene[18]

- Benzene is a highly flammable colorless to light yellow chemical.

- Benzene is liquid at room temperature.

- Benzene comes from both industrial and natural sources:
    - Natural Sources include emissions from volcanoes, forest fires, crude oil and cigarette smoke.
    - Outdoor air contains low levels of benzene from tobacco smoke, automobile service stations, exhaust from motor vehicles and industrial emissions.
    - Vapors or gases from products that contain benzene such as glues, paints, furniture wax, and detergents.

- Benzene Carries a Health Hazard 2 Warning (Slightly Hazardous).

- Benzene may cause adverse reproductive effects and birth defects. May affect genetic material (mutagenic). May cause cancer (tumorigenic, leukemia) Human: passes the placental barrier, detected in maternal milk.

- Benzene ranks in the top 20 chemicals for production volume for a wide range of chemicals as well as motor fuel:
  - More than half of benzene is used for production of polymers and plastics.
  - 20% for production of resins and adhesives.
  - 10% for the production of nylon fibers for textiles and plastics.
  - The remaining amounts of benzene are used for the production of detergents, drugs, dyes, explosives, rubbers, lubricants, and pesticides.[19]

- IARC (International Agency for Research on Cancer) Carcinogenicity Classification is A-1: Confirmed Carcinogen The IARC first reported benzene in this classification in 1987.

- ACGIH (American Conference of Governmental Industrial Hygienist) classification of benzene in Group 1: Proven Carcinogen in 2006.

- EPA (Environmental Protection Agency) classified benzene as A1 "Confirmed Carcinogen" in 2006.

- DHHS (U.S. Department of Health and Human Services) has determined that benzene causes cancer in humans in 2013.

- NTP (U.S Department of Toxicology Program) classification as a Group K: the K is for "Known to be Human Carcinogen" in 2005.

- ATSDR (Agency for Toxic Substance and Disease Registry) states:
  - Breathing very high levels of benzene can result in death.
  - High levels of benzene can cause:
    - Drowsiness
    - Dizziness
    - Rapid heart rate

- Headaches
- Tremors
- Confusion
- Unconsciousness
- Long term exposure causes effects are on bone marrow and can cause anemia and leukemia.
- Eating or Drinking food containing high levels of benzene can cause:
  - Vomiting
  - Irritation of the stomach
  - Dizziness
  - Sleepiness
  - Convulsions
  - Rapid heart rate
  - Death[20]

- CDC (Centers for Disease Control) claims there is no specific antidote for benzene poisoning.

- EPA (Environmental Protection Agency) has found benzene in at least 1000 out of 1684 of the sites identified as hazardous and on the National Priority List. The National Priority List is a list of the known releases of hazardous substances in the United States.

- OSHA (Occupational Safety & Health Administration) Toxicity Summary:[21]
  - OSHA Identification and Use: as a starter material in manufacturing other chemicals, including detergents, pesticides, plastics, and resins, synthetic rubber, aviation fuel, pharmaceuticals, dye, explosives, PCB gasoline, flavors and perfumes, paints and coatings, nylon intermediates, and photographic chemicals.
  - OSHA Long term health effects of exposure of a year or more affects:
    - Bone marrow and a decrease in red cells, leading to anemia.

- Can cause excessive bleeding and can affect the immune system, increasing chance of infection.
- Long term exposure to high levels of benzene in the air can cause leukemia, cancer of the blood forming organs.

Toluene and benzene are the most elementary and fundamental of petroleum chemicals and are what the industrial world calls "starter material" or "feed stock" for organic synthesis.[22] **Chemists use the word "organic" to designate all substances containing carbon, but not all things containing carbon are life enhancing, some of these carbons include deadly poisons. Benzene is such a carbon.**

Organic synthesis simply means taking something from nature and creating *a synthetic version with toluene or benzene as the molecular building material*. The end result is a fake **petrochemical** product based on something from nature. This terminology confused me for years and maybe confusing others today.

Structure vs. Formula

In organic chemistry the structure is as important as the formula.[23] The human body responds to the structure primarily. Scientists write and rewrite chemical formulas using the mother solvent molecules as the base structure for any given modern product from shampoo to chemotherapy.

These formulas of organic synthesis for recreating mother nature can change on paper but within your body, your cells *know* that it's a structure made of the benzene molecule.

Your body is intelligent.

The bottom line for your cells is the structure of the molecule. Your cells want and need structures that are the right size for the human cell receptor site. Like a perfect size key for a lock;

structure and size matters to our cells.

On the molecular level the benzene molecule is clumsy, the wrong size, missing the vital force,[24] with incorrectly placed outer electrons, or valance electrons[25] and having a synthetic structure that the human cell's elegant receptor sites finds insulting.

This wrong size **causes damage** to the **elegant receptor site**. The benzene structures are just too big, like a pair of shoes that are two sizes too big. The shoe and the chemical structure just don't fit and can make you fall flat on your molecular face!

Remember the following about products in our environment that are made from the mother solvent:

If you smell it,
it's within your lungs.

If you rub it on,
it's absorbed by your skin.

If you eat it,
it's consumed by your digestive system.

It's now within your body,
along with all its effects... known and unknown.

Modern medicine is an industry built on chemical compounds synthetically created by toluene/methyl benzene and benzene and chlorine structures (as well other structures of mold and bacteria). It's worth repeating, in basic organic chemistry, structure is just as essential as composition.

In the September 2011 edition of Harvard *Women's Health Watch* states: "The term bio identical doesn't have an exact medical definition," and further states that "any custom-compounded hormones have effects in the body, they're drugs." Although people may believe the marketing term "bio-identical" is safer, my body knows the truth. My body sees right past the chemical impostor and sees the true structure, and knows it's not bio-identical. Is your body recognizing the impostor? Are you being robbed of your vitality by a benzene structure poser being marketed to you as "bio identical"?

My last ER visit resulted in a near heart attack from an IV of steroids and this was the day I became officially diagnosed with Chemical Intolerance. I was given a very strict warning by the doctor to never have any steroid medication again. I was warned I would not survive it. I would later learn that steroids are organic synthesis of flowers.[26]

Many Compounds are Based in Petrochemicals

Benzodiazepine is another offspring of the mother solvent is also fondly known by those who fight its addiction as "benzos". Benzodiazepine known as "this class of psychoactive drugs whose core chemical structure is the fusion of a benzene ring and a diazepine ring."[27] (Some have the opinion that the pharmaceutical use of benzene and toluene are a great service to mankind. In my opinion the petrochemical's core structure produces dire consequences for all of us and dire consequences for our collective future generations.)

Gasoline is an example of how these two basic components of crude oil are used. Toluene and benzene are mixed with xylene to create gasoline.[28] When gasoline goes through a combustion engine the resulting exhaust contains unburnt carbon molecules of benzene, toluene, and xylene, called carbon-monoxide. Carbon-monoxide poisoning is a type of fatal air poisoning caused by these unburnt molecules.

Nail Polish is a blend of toluene and benzene disguised as nitrocellulose, dibutyl phthalate (DBP), formaldehyde, and ethyl acetate and is applied to the tips of our our fingers and toes which is also the tips of our nervous system, and the end of some of our meridian channels. Removing the polish gives this area of the body another concentrated dose of toluene and benzene. Giving up my painted toenails was another sacrifice I made many decades ago, after I noticed the connection of the polish and splitting skin around the nails and feeling weakened in general after applying it and smelling it. This is how I begin to see that the mother solvent's offsprings have many disguises under many names. To learn more about your beauty products see Resources.

Nitroglycerin is a petrochemical compound used as a common heart medication as well as an explosive. This drug is a mixture of toluene treated with nitric and sulfuric acids. During this process trinitrotoluene is produced, also known as TNT or nitroglycerin.

There are over seven million (7,000,000!) organically synthesized compounds that have been made in a lab with feed stock of benzene and toluene rather than grown from nature. You can begin to see how things get scary, fast! These benzene based petrochemicals are in our medicine, food, beauty products, body washes, toothpaste, make up, deodorants and hundreds of other places you would never suspect.

Benzene and toluene are the basic molecular structures used to create fake or synthetic compounds such as pharmaceuticals, dyes, detergents, solvents, pesticides, lubricants, and explosives. There's synthetic cloth, synthetic food, synthetic medicine, synthetic vitamins, synthetic minerals... the list goes on and on.

Your chemical sensitivity could be due to one of these _organic synthesized_ products. Products with a base molecular structure of toluene or benzene masked under many assumed names.

In my opinion toluene and benzene released from boiling crude oil, coal tar or fracking shale, do not belong within the human body, ever. Science tells us that exposure to toluene and benzene effects the nervous system. I have first hand experience explained within the chapters of this book. The effects of exposure to an affected nervous system are dysfunctional and not life enhancing.

The following is a short list of ingredients that you may be using without realizing you are using toluene and benzene feed stock based consumer goods. I also provide MSDS, Materials Safety Data Sheets, at the end of the book on each of these common ingredients.

Diethanolamine or DEA[29] is an ingredient found in:

- Body Washes
- Bubble Baths
- Conditioners
- Cosmetics
- Dish Detergents
- Lotions
- Laundry
- Shampoos

It's an emulsifier, a thickener, and it makes foam. In pharmaceuticals it's used as a raw material in the production of:

- Antihistamines
- Anti-malaria
- Antibiotics
- Local Anesthetics
- Antidepressants
- Muscle Relaxants

Commonly used ingredients that may contain DEA.[30]

- Cocamide DEA
- Coamide DEA
- Cocamide MEA
- DEA-Cetyl Phosphate
- DEA Oleth-3 Phosphate
- Lauramide DEA

- Linoleamide MEA
- Myristamide DEA
- Oleamide DEA
- Stearamide MEA
- TEA-Lauryl Sulfate
- Triethanolamine

- Diethanolamine now carries a Health Hazard warning of (3) Extreme Danger, major injury likely.
- Diethanolamine had been in the past listed as a Health Hazard of (1).

Propylene Glycol[1] has a wide range of industrial uses. It stops things from dying out such as:

- Anti-freeze
- Baby Wipes
- Brake and Hydraulic Fluids
- Cosmetics
- De-icer
- Deodorants
- Floor Wax
- Laundry Detergent
- Shampoos
- Soft Chewy Dog Food Morsels
- Tobacco
- Toothpaste
- Paints and Coatings
- Processed Foods

- Propylene Glycol may be listed in ingredient lists as a humectants.
- Propylene Glycol is an irritant and a permeator.
- Propylene Glycol may be toxic to central nervous system.
- Propylene Glycol may produce target organ damage.
- Propylene Glycol carries a Health Hazard of "Generally regarded as safe" on the GRAS list.

Sodium Lauryl Sulfate or SLS[32] or Sodium Laureth Sulfate SLES is a surfactant. Surfactants are used to break down the surface tension of water.

- Some industrial uses are:

  - Body Washes
  - Car Wash Detergents
  - Concrete Floor Cleaners
  - Detergents
  - Engine Cleaner
  - Used to De-foam in Food Processing
  - Food Degreasers
  - Toothpaste
  - Shampoos

- There is an ongoing debate over SLS and SLES. Over the years I have read numerous websites saying it does not cause cancer. My experience begs to differ. For a chemically intolerant person it's all about the benzene structure that SLS is built upon.
- The original plant structure of sodium lauryl sulfate is coconuts, the organic synthesis version is built with a benzene molecule. Remember, *organic* in this context does not mean "grown without chemicals."
- Repeated or prolonged exposure to this substance can produce target organ damage as well as produce a deterioration of health by an accumulation in one or many human organs.
- Additionally the E in SLES is ethylene oxide another possible trouble maker for the MCS individual.
  - Ethylene oxide is used in industry to make the other chemicals less harsh by a process called ethoxylation. This process is used to make laundry detergent and other personal care products such as shampoo, toothpaste and sterilization of medical supplies, etc.

- Ethylene oxide has a Hazard Warning of 3.
- There is a byproduct of ethoxylation that is a suspect in cancer. This byproduct is 1,4-dioxane.
- Sodium Lauryl Sulfate carries a Health Hazard: 2, slightly hazardous, temporary or minor injury.

It's the accumulation of benzene molecules through the use of many chemically based products throughout the day that was creating stress on my kidneys and liver. If I use soap in a public bathroom I have muscle cramps in my hands. That's the benzene molecules setting off my inner alarm system. This seemingly innocent ingredient is everywhere. We're saturated in SLS and SLES unless as chemically sensitive people we begin to read all labels and only use products that do not include these poisons.

tert-Butylhydroquinone or TBHQ[33] several different MSDS give this chemical a hefty warning. TBHQ or tert-Butylhydroquinone, is used as a food additive and food antioxidant.

- tert-Butylhydroquinone or TBHQ is another petrochemical found in common restaurant oil and it sets off a chemical intolerance episode of epic proportions for me.
- tert-Butylhydroquinone is found in animal feeds, cosmetics and personal care, edible fats and flavorings. This chemical is also found in microwave popcorn and other things that are designed to blow up... like bombs. Yes, this is a bomb making ingredient and your body may also find it highly insulting and rude!
- Other names for TBHQ related chemicals:
  - tert-butylhydroquinone
  - tertiary butylhydroquinone
  - butylated hydroxyanisol
  - 2-tert-Butyl-1
  - 4-benzenediol
- tert-Butylhydroquinone has Potential Health Effects if swallowed, inhaled, or absorbed through the skin is harmful and the target organs are blood, liver, respiratory system,

eyes, and skin.
- 0.02% by volume is allowed in our food or just over 75 drops per every five gallon container of oil.
- Health Hazard: (2) Slightly Hazardous, temporary or minor injury

Some people innocently believe that we're protected from harsh chemicals. This is just naivete. In 1938 the FDA grandfathered in a list of ingredients generally regarded as safe known as the GRAS list (Generally Recognized As Safe) for personal care and food. In 1938, little was known about the long term effects of any of these chemicals. Decades later, in 1973 the FDA began a review of all items of the GRAS list. Some items were removed from the "safe" list and some items were given interim status on "a not so safe list." That interim status has expired. Now, over thirty years later many of the interim status ingredients such as BHT, (which by the way is now determined harmful by other country's standards) are still in the American food supply.

When Natural Isn't Natural

Do not be fooled by labels making claims of "Natural". There are no standards or oversight for "Natural" like there is for "USDA Certified Organic." I have seen "Natural" on labels that include petroleum products. A nurse actually told me years ago that crude oil comes from the earth and is considered natural. I was dumbfounded and went looking for the truth myself.

According to the FDA[34] website; "From a food science perspective, it's difficult to define a food product that is "natural" because the food has probably been processed and is no longer the product of the earth. That said, the FDA has not developed a definition for use of the term "natural" or its derivatives. However, the agency has not objected to the use of the term "natural" if the food does not contain added color, artificial flavors, or synthetic substances."

This is confusing since most "natural" flavorings are extracted with chemicals from the mother solvent, and considered... natural.

Under the Code of Federal Regulations the definition of natural flavor is: "the essential oil, oleo-resin, essence or extractive, protein hydrolysate or enzymolysis, which contains the flavoring constituents derived from:

- A spice, fruit, or fruit juice.
- A vegetable or vegetable juice.
- An edible yeast, herb, bark, bud, root, leaf, or similar plant material.
- Meat, seafood, poultry, eggs, or dairy products
- Fermentation Products
- "Whose significant function is flavoring rather than nutritional" (21CFR101.22).

University of Minnesota, professor of food science and nutrition, Gary Reineccius says, "both artificial and natural flavors may be created in the lab by "flavorists" by blending either natural or synthetic chemicals[35] to create the desired flavorings."[36]

In an email clarifying his statement, Professor Reineccius explained that essential oils can create the desired flavor as well as the synthetic chemicals. Synthetic flavorings are not stronger, better or more desirable for flavorings.

Looking for the organic label is one way to take back control of what you're eating, or does it? The USDA Organic National Program regulates crops, livestock, and agricultural products certified to the United States Department of Agriculture's organic standards; "Synthetic fertilizers, sewage, sludge, irradiation, and genetic engineering may not be used." However, be aware that as of May 2004 the USDA[37] will no longer monitor or police organic label claims on what they have defined as non-food or non-agricultural products, like body care products, vitamins, nutritional supplements, fertilizers, and even seafood.

The USDA is placing this task on the FDA, an agency who has declared it does not regulate organic.[38]

Following the guidelines of the USDA[39] website continues to clarify "natural": "The USDA requires that meat and poultry and egg products labeled as "Natural" must be minimally processed and contain no artificial ingredients. However, the natural label does not include any standards regarding practice of "natural" flavors. Natural flavors can still contain solvents, emulsifiers and preservatives; all of which come under a category of "incidental additives" and are <u>not</u> required to be disclosed by the food manufacturers. The Environmental Working Group reports: "Flavor extracts and food ingredients that have been derived from genetically engineered crops may also be labeled "natural" because the FDA has not fully defined what that term "natural" means." In other words don't trust anything labeled "natural" on the front and turn it around and read the entire ingredient list. Until greed is gone from our society, it's best to reject "Natural" and go for "Certified Organic", it's the only way to be sure in these United States of America, for anyone desiring to avoid chemicals in their food.

There are other ingredients in products that you may be using every day that are not listed above. If you want to know more about the ingredients listed on a product; I highly encourage you to do your own research as I have done. Many things available today have not been thoroughly tested; therefore it requires you to be an informed consumer and know what you are consuming.

Avoid listening to mainstream media for your scientific research information. Conduct your own research. This is especially important if you're sick, someone you love is sick, or if you have little ones trusting you to protect them. Only you have the power of your mind to protect you.

Only in recent decades has science addressed some false beliefs that have been presented as fact for decades. The first false belief is that the body has a special mechanism that switches on in the presence of toxic chemicals to break them down and usher them out of the body. Only recently has science begun to grasp that the original offending toxins are not broken down to less toxic substances but rather they create a synergistic horror story for the metabolic processes of the body's systems.

Another shattered belief is that animals and humans react the same and metabolize toxic substances in similar ways. Decades of animal testing has led researchers to know the facts; that humans are elegantly more complex than mice, and the results from animal testing through the decades has been misleading and inaccurate. Shortly after this truth came to light The 1987, 2004, and 2007 IARC (International Agency for Research on Cancer) reports placed benzene in a Carcinogenicity Classifications. The National Toxicology Program classification of benzene was placed in Group K "Known to be Human Carcinogen" in 2005.

Despite the currently held belief that petrochemicals are excreted from the body completely, I'm one hundred percent certain that these toxins are not fully excreted from the human body without help. My own experience supports the theory that a body has a storage system for its own protection. My many years of observing myself and others support my theory that these chemicals and other foreign elements like heavy metals, stay trapped within the body's fat, jaw bone, feet, and in layers of the skin. It's storage is also evidenced in the swelling of the spleen, liver, lymph nodes, endocrine glands and breasts.

Today, I believe a new false belief is being circulated that those of us with Multiple Chemical Sensitivity carry a genetic mutation. How can human DNA carry a genetic mutation for something developed long after humanity's arrival? How can you have a mutation for something that didn't exist before our DNA? I assure you mankind has existed long before benzene and toluene were extracted from the heart of mother earth and boiled. The benzene structure is the aberration, not us.

I see many people walking around with swollen abdomens and I ask myself if that's because of worms, leaky gut, or from enlarged liver, kidneys, or spleen due to benzene exposure? As I talk with people I learn (without prompting) that they're on medication for the suppression of symptoms due to ill organs such as thyroid and pancreas. As a chemically sensitive individual, whenever I took medications some of my organs were either swelling or being knocked out of homeostasis and showing signs of dysfunction. I am proof that ingesting more medication is not what's needed by the chemically sensitive body. The body needs help from other sources.

It needs to be heard.

It needs __TRUE__ healing support.

<u>Chapter Seven</u>

A Quantum Turn of Events

"Strange is our situation here on Earth. Each of us comes for a short visit, not knowing why, yet sometimes seeming to a divine purpose... There is one thing we do know: that man is here for the sake of other men."
~Albert Einstein~

A full understanding of the dangers of toluene had not been reached as I continued to naively remove BHT from my life, and fully engage my career as a theatrical scene designer. One day I used surplus spray paint on a stage piece, spraying outside in a well ventilated area. Eight hours later my body reacted with shocking symptoms. I woke up to the news that I had been in a coma for three days, a spinal tap had revealed **lead** poisoning. Because of my toluene allergy the doctors had chosen to take a wait and see approach. This additional burden of lead into my system forever changed my career path and my life as an artist.

My health demanded that I remove myself from theater stage design and stage craft chemicals. My marriage would eventually crumble and I found myself a single mother and a I.A.T.S.E. (International Alliance of Theatrical Stage Employees) freelance stagehand. I would work on many different types of stage productions from trade show installation as well as rock and roll concerts, eventually I was able to move full time into costumes and film making. In my spare time I did research to learn more about the mysterious toluene.

Armed with the knowledge I gained from my research I continued to manage my exposure to products made with petrochemicals. I thought I knew how to give myself healing support as I made adjustments in my life as a divorced single mom and freelance film maker. My job choices included less potential for exposure to petrochemicals.

Years later I remarried. It was so exciting to find love with someone who understood and supported my needs as a Multiple Chemical Sensitive individual. My life became more fun and interesting. I still had challenges though.

At 37 years old I became pregnant with my second child. In my fifth month of pregnancy I was asphyxiated with diesel fumes! Working in the film industry is not easy and can be dangerous at times. On this particular show I was working with someone so careless, they parked a large, exhaust creating, generator next to my truck (in the movies and TV you work out of converted semi-trucks). This placed the air intake of my truck at the exhaust out flow of the generator.

Invisible carbon monoxide was pumped into the truck where I was working. If not for one of my astute wardrobe crew members pulling me out into the fresh air, I would have died along with my unborn child. Instead I spent the afternoon on an oxygen tank with a paramedic checking my blood pressure. I was worried about my baby but unfortunately the paramedic couldn't reassure me, and my doctor explained that it's unknown what happens to a fetus exposed to carbon monoxide.

My baby, a son, was born full term and healthy. This hospital visit was shorter than my first. The thirteen years between babies had softened the rules in the maternity ward. My doctor and I had a long term relationship and he thought he understood my chemical issues. It surprised him when I didn't respond to the anesthetic as expected, but it all worked out in the end and everyone went home happy and healthy.

My beautiful son grew and thrived first on breast milk and later from the bottle. He made it to six months old and then demanded more solid food. He was an eating machine, banging on the tray of the highchair for another bite. It was a very funny sight to see this little guy eating multiple jars of baby food at each sitting.

I was happily enjoying the moment, unaware that my sweet journey through life would soon take an abrupt turn when one summer afternoon exposure to paint sent me to the ER. The attending doctor prescribed a steroid IV. As I faded away, that was my last memory as my body rejected the offending substance. When I awoke the doctor told me I was lucky to be alive.

I would leave the hospital with a new medical diagnosis, "Chemical Intolerant." The ER doctor sternly advised me to avoid all petroleum based chemicals and to never allow anyone to give me steroid medication. The doctor's concern was genuine as he told me I may not survive the next round of steroid medication, which is the standard of care for the MCS individual. I will say it was a hair rising ER visit and I took the doctor's advice seriously. I have children who need their mother!

After the steroid medication fiasco I became aware of swelling in my arms and thighs. It had started that day in the ER and had not gone down. It also seemed like I was continuing to get bigger. A medical checkup and basic medical tests came back normal. Additional testing came back normal as well. Again, another doctor dismisses my inexplicable, to them, symptoms.

A friend was convinced the swelling and excess weight was a nutritionally based problem. She introduced me to a researcher working with supplements and taking readings on a little computer-like device that was being referred to as "bio-resonance." The sessions were very expensive so I could only budget myself a few. These sessions did seem to help me. At that point I started searching for anything that was referred to as "bio-resonance."

Trusting Mother's Intuition

We celebrated our son's fifth birthday. He was a healthy, happy child until a few days later when his stomachaches began. He would eat and then cry for hours and then whimper about how bad his stomach hurt. This went on for several months every day, after every meal.

I promptly called our pediatrician who was out of the office and the physician on call didn't understand the severity of the problem. This doctor gave up on diagnosing our son after one simple blood test did not reveal an ulcer. This meant there were no referrals to a specialist, just another round of blood tests looking for ulcers. The doctor prescribed drugs for his painful crying and screaming. These medications made his stomach hurt more and nothing stopped the pain.

My concern for for my son's health increased, which I didn't think possible. Doctors and their medications weren't able to help us. I went searching for the researcher that had the "bio-resonance" tool and nutritional information that had helped me. Unfortunately, he could not be located. It became critical for me to research nutrition and teach myself about the digestive system. My mother's intuition was assuring me that a solution would be found.

My son had dark circles under his eyes, was not gaining weight, and not growing. Abruptly he started losing weight and the doctor suggested cancer testing. I knew my son didn't have cancer. My intuition was telling me that there was another answer. This doctor wasn't using critical thinking. He was jumping to conclusions, in my opinion.

How does someone go from eating one meal without a stomachache and then have such terrible stomach pains the next 100 meals? Since something similar had happened to me with my chemical sensitivity and PMS symptoms I assumed his problems ran along the same lines. I asked for another round of testing this time for more nutritional type markers. The doctor assured me he would request these tests and then failed to do so.

I fired that doctor.

Instead of spinning into a frenzied action seeking out a new doctor my intuition kicked in stronger than ever. I felt an inner need to be still. With this inner stillness I turned my full attention to God and listened for the answer. I prayed and affirmed that everything in my life was a blessing and somehow so was my son's stomach aches.

The doctors didn't know and only one force in this world did know, and that was the Creator. So, I returned to my childhood heroes, Baby Jesus, God, and the little moron. The secret in unlocking this blessing was faith in action.

I began meditating more frequently. One day I felt the pull of my intuition to attend a meditation presentation at a bookstore. Attending that presentation began a series of connections that lead to the synchronization of events resulting in my son's healing.

The Lady in Red

Valentina sat all in red and as cool as a glass of lemonade. She was the meditation presenter. What happens next is all divine.

Valentina, the meditation facilitator asked why we were attending the class. When I shared that for me it was about my little boy. She explained that she had something that would help him. Valentina had a bio-resonance device. She explained that this device measured endocrine system reactions and could recreate the frequency as a homeopathic remedy.

It identified that his problem was the pancreas and *petroleum chemicals*. Valentina looked at me and in all sincerity asked me if my child played at gas stations.

"Of course not!" I exclaimed. "However, could it be from *his gestation*?" I asked her.

"Certainly." she replied.

So it all happened to him in utero... now I know what happens if a fetus is asphyxiated; their pancreas development gets interrupted by these toxins and later in life they can't digest their food!

My son's story has a happy ending. After three days on the homeopathic formula created for him by Valentina, he woke up in the morning and asked for and ate an entire bowl of oatmeal. We all waited for the pain to hit him. To our relief there was No Pain. He ate a second bowl of oatmeal and then some applesauce. There was NO PAIN.

We experienced a miracle!

Our gratitude was immeasurable. We were given the answer so effortlessly and it ended this excruciating experience. It would take a few more sessions with Valentina before our child eventually remained pain free and began to thrive. His little body had been heard and it responded by beginning the return to homeostasis. His body had innate healing abilities and with true healing support the impossible was made possible.

It would be years before I would fully realize what we had *actually* experienced with our son's miracle healing. At the time overwhelmed with gratitude, I was blinded by personal joy, I didn't see that we had been placed at the cusp of Tomorrow's Medicine... a medicine born from quantum physics.

<u>Chapter Eight</u>

Death: The Final Symptom

*"I believe in intuitions and inspirations... I sometimes <u>feel</u> that I
am right. I do not <u>know</u> that I am right."*
~Albert Einstein~

When my next chemically induced health trauma occurred
my inner guidance failed me, or so it seemed. The long awaited
Michael Mann movie remake of the popular TV series, *Miami
Vice*, had started shooting. I was hired to prepare costumes for
male extras. I was expecting to enjoy this job and it to be fun as I
was an original member of the costume crew for the original TV
series and I expected to see some old friends on the job for the
feature film. During preparations for a large crowd scene, I was
exposed to chemicals from the special effects department. Fumes
came through the air conditioning vents into my work
environment.

This was a devastating event for me!

Once again I was poisoned. As I tried to decide how to
handle this new crisis my intuition suddenly was telling me <u>not</u> to
go to the emergency room. Remember, my last dramatic ER visit
included the terrible reaction to steroid medication. That ER
physician impressed upon me not to ever have another steroid shot,
IV, or pill as my heart would not make it.

I heard his kind stern warning, "It will be the end of you if
you do."

Every molecule of my body implored me to listen to my
intuition.

As a result of my chemical exposure that day I would spend
the night on the bathroom floor alternating between being

conscious and unconscious. When I was conscious I had simultaneous vomiting and diarrhea. As I was on the bathroom floor I heard the comforting voice of my guru who had passed away a decade before, advising me to, "Listen to your intuition, it will save your life one day." My intuition screamed, "THIS IS THAT DAY."

One of the consequences of choosing not to go to the ER was that I was not able to file a worker's compensation claim. In addition to not receiving insurance coverage for the injury, I also did not receive compensation for any lost wages. People often assume that I received some form of compensation for this catastrophic injury. I did not.

Being true to myself I recognized this illness as a blessing. I just had to be like the little moron and dig through all the pony manure. After a month I was still very sick from the chemical exposure which was slowly poisoning me. My abdomen, upper arms and thighs were swelling. Even though I was barely able to eat I was swollen as if I was stuffing my face. At the same time I tried to pretend I was not sick. I was failing at faking it.

Chemical poisoning robs you of your energy. Toluene affects the nervous system. My head was full of mucus and I had no gumption. Another problem with chemical poisoning is that you don't look sick until you are near death. I felt near death but no one was hearing me. Since I had opted not to go to the emergency room my family assumed I was exhausted and I would snap out of it soon. I didn't.

Everything I did was an effort. Everything was exhausting. If I made it to work I had to continually lie down and rest. My co-workers knew something was wrong as they knew me as a work horse and a non-stop machine. Instead I was getting worse with each job. One day of work took me two weeks to recover from the fatigue.

My daughter and her family moved in with us at the same time. Our world was upside down as we recovered from hurricane damage and incorporated my daughter, her husband, and their brand new baby girl into our lives. Having my daughter and my first beautiful granddaughter at home meant everything to me. I wanted to savor every moment, but I couldn't. I was just too sick.

I started calling Valentina, the lady in red who had been so much help with my son. After many attempts I couldn't find her and finally gave up. Finding out more about the technology Valentina used became my new obsession. In spite of the internet and Google I found little information on anything regarding 'bio-resonance' equipment.

Once again I surrendered to faith in my intuition, knowing that the information I needed would come to me. However, when I could no longer hold myself up on the toilet or the sink and I was forced to surrendered to the bathroom floor, in that moment I was sure that I was going to leave this life like Elvis.[2]

PART THREE:

The Solutions

I survived that night. I survived what a friend and an acquaintance would later die of; liver failure. My friend didn't have the arsenal of knowledge that I have and that I'm now sharing with you. The following section is my current collection of solutions.

The body needs to be heard.

It needs true healing support. So many of us are looking for just that, but what does "that" look like? How does the body get to be heard? How can you help your body if all medicine is made from the very thing making you sick?

Are you frustrated? I feel your frustration. I was dumbfounded at how bad the toxicity picture really is. It was important for me to continue following my intuition. Now over three decades later, I'm still alive. I'm over sixty years and not on any medication. I feel vibrant and mentally focused. Sadly, I cannot say the same for several friends who followed conventional medical wisdom.

<u>Chapter Nine</u>

Leaf Me Forever

"Truth tends to present itself modestly and in simple garb."
~Albert Einstein~

My first non-traditional solution was introduced to me around 1996. Like most people at the time I had no idea what an Essential Oil was. Today more and more people are being introduced to the powerful healing that can be attained with the use of Essential Oils. For those who may not have had a full introduction to caring for oneself with these wonderful gifts of nature I will give a brief introduction.

As a child I loved the story of the three wise men and their gifts. These three gifts of the Magi given to the baby Jesus were actual gifts of Essential Oils. When the ancient tombs of the Pharaohs were opened, thousands of years after their creation, they were filled with golden treasures; but the large urns containing Essential Oils had been robbed. One urn left behind by the ancient grave robbers contained viable Essential Oil, carbon dated at over 3000 years old.

What was it about these ancient oils that would mean more to thieves than fortunes of gold, and kings would offer as gifts?

What's Better than Gold?

Essential Oil!

- Essential Oil[1] is the life blood of a plant.

- Essential Oil is any of a large class of volatile odoriferous oils of vegetable origin that give plants their characteristic odors and often other properties.

- Essential Oil is obtained from various parts of the plants such as flowers, leaves, or bark.

- Essential Oils are derived by steam distillation, expression, or extraction, that are usually mixtures of compounds (as aldehydes or esters).

- Essential Oil is used often in the form of essences in perfumes, flavorings, and pharmaceutical preparations.

- Essential Oil also called ethereal oil or volatile oil.

- They do not compare to fatty oil or fixed oil.

- Pharmaceutical grade essential oils may be organically synthesized from the mother solvent.

- Essential Oil is different from vegetable oils like corn, peanut, soybean, or canola oil. These "fixed oils" are actually vegetable *fats* which can clog pores.

Essential Oils are not fatty oils, nor fixed oils, but rather the plant's unique liquid intelligences coming together as a collage. They contain thousands of components and all these ingredients delicately dancing in harmony. Essential Oil of herbs are up to one hundred times stronger than their dried powder counterpart. Trees, shrubs, leaves, flowers, roots and seeds all contain many aromatic liquids and solids that can be distilled into a vapor. The vapor collected contains the plant's <u>most powerful healing attributes</u>. This vapor is returned back to liquid and it's the essential liquid or "oil" of the plant.

The plant kingdom has an innate intelligence, as does the human body. An example of this innate intelligence would be your immune system kicking into high gear when your body is under attack from germs. The plant's subtle innate intelligence has properties that protect the plant from germs; and other disease causing microbes. Some plant's protective properties have antibacterial, antiviral, or antifungal elements.

Capturing these delicate components is one important aspect in the *ART* of therapeutic grade Essential Oil production. From the seed of the plant to how it's grown, harvested and distilled affects the levels of certain components (or intelligence) that's in the resulting Essential Oil. To be a *therapeutic grade Essential Oil,* the levels of certain ingredients, components, and constituents must be within certain ranges and nothing else. It's only then that the oil will deliver its highest intelligence, its most valuable properties into every cell of your body.

Therapeutic Essential Oils affected me in a positive way. Their effects upon my cells were life changing for me.

History supports me. Essential Oils have been used medicinally by ancient healers throughout mankind's history to kill bacteria, fungi, and viruses. Additional value comes from fragrance to lift moods, release emotional blocks, and create an ambiance for love. Ancient healers also knew Essential Oils were versatile in their ability to stimulate and regenerate nerves, carry nutrients, and oxygenate cells. Even the ancient tomb raiders knew the true treasure was the Essential Oils.

Killing Migraines in Their Tracks

My introduction to therapeutic grade Essential Oils was with the versatile and widely used peppermint oil. One day at work, around 1996, I started getting the symptoms of a migraine headache. Typically, I keep any personal medical issues to myself as people start offering aspirin and more. It just takes too much energy to explain my issues, but this day was different.

I turned to my crew and sighed "I'm getting a migraine headache and I'm not in the mood for work today."

Prepared for the usual kindly drug offerings, I was surprised when a co-worker and friend, Heather came forward with an **alternative**.

"I have something that might help." Heather said, "It's something different, something natural from a plant."

She was holding a tiny little bottle, taking my hand she placed a single drop of peppermint oil on my thumb. She then had me stick my thumb into my mouth and push it up on the roof of my mouth (like a baby sucking his thumb). In less than a minute I felt this surge of energy up through my head and the rush pushed the headache away. I was in <u>love</u>!

Migraine headaches are terrible, they can last for days and force you into a quiet, dark room with pain and vomiting. Unless you've had one, you have no idea how bad they are. Let alone how hard it is to go through life with the looming threat of a migraine. For me that one drop of peppermint was a miracle. I have not been without it since.

My Surprising Results

After that incredible experience with peppermint oil, I began another learning journey, this time I researched the difference between "regular" and "therapeutic grade" Essential Oils. The peppermint oil my friend Heather offered me was from a company some of you may already be familiar with called Young Living Essential Oils (YLEO).

Young Living Essential Oils is a family owned company founded by D. Gary Young. Gary survived a near fatal accident leaving him paralyzed from the neck down. After years of recovery he came to understand the tremendous capabilities of the body and its innate powers of healing. Today Gary Young has reclaimed his ability to walk and has dedicated decades to research and cultivation of Essential Oils from seed to seal, bringing back to the people authentic therapeutic grade Essential Oils.

Young Living's Essential Oils in the past were labeled

therapeutic grade based on world standards and guidelines, as set forth by the International Standards Organization (ISO)[2] and Association French Normalization Regulation Committee (a European agency whose acronym is AFNOR).[3]

Everywhere in the world, except the United States, Essential Oils labeled 100 % Pure Therapeutic Grade have met the standards of the ISO and have a certificate on record from AFNOR. To create the AFNOR certification the world's finest scientists and doctors in organic chemistry worked together to create standards for Essential Oils. Doctors such as Dr. Herve Casabianca, considered the world expert in the science of Essential Oils. Dr. Casabianca, holds a doctoral degree in organic chemistry and is an expert in the isotopic and chromatographic analysis used in the dissection of an Essential Oil. Unfortunately, in today's world of pollution some unsavory molecules are slipping past current detection methods.

With today's environmental challenges of radiation, pollution, as well as more sophisticated organic synthesis of essentially everything of plant origin, more sophisticated testing methods for Essential Oils are required. Young Living is working to bring higher standards and guidelines for therapeutic grade oils in the United States.

In the United States inferior oils abound with labels such as "natural", "organic", "pure", "food grade" or "pharmaceutical grade." Sadly, the uninformed consumer runs the risk of using Essential Oils that are inferior synthetic versions created from petrochemicals or adulterated with petrochemical extenders. I can, assure you that most will give you less than desirable results and could possibly be dangerous for those with multiple chemical sensitivities and chemical intolerance.

As I mentioned earlier, in the United States there are no standards for Essential Oils. Gary Young is working to that end. For now it's up to you to do your due diligence. For the suppliers it's up to their good manufacturing practices and ethics. If you decide you want to try Essential Oils for yourself, I can only recommend Young Living Therapeutic Grade Essential Oils at this time, as I'm unaware of any other companies with the standards necessary to protect the Multiple Chemical Sensitive and Chemical Intolerant individuals.

It's important to know and trust your supplier of Essential Oils.

Therapeutic grade Essential Oils are structurally compatible with the body. These Essential Oils are closest in structure to the human blood and are easily assimilated by the body. Their plant origins are the correct structure and the right constituents that your body needs, craves and desires.

With the right constituents and <u>no other structures of pesticides, fertilizer or other toxic pollutants in the mix</u>... these molecular structures will be a perfect fit for starved dirty cells! They fit because they were designed to fit.

It's a perfect fit, like your car into your garage, an airplane into a hanger, a comfortable sized shoe unto your foot. They fit because they were designed to fit. The airplane would not fit into the garage of your house without breaking down the walls and creating damage. A car would easily fit into the airplane hanger, but there would be much space left over, unused, wasted space.

Comprehending <u>the importance of the small and subtle</u> with simple structures is one step into **Tomorrow's Medicine**. Your cells are precise storage structures of intelligent energy, designed to interact with only certain sizes, shapes, intelligences and constituents. Anything else causes waste or cell damage at the worst.

Throughout my life I've had to be budget minded instead of quality minded. Once long ago, I tried an inferior, cheap clove oil being sold by a well known and respected American supplement company. The intense burning and redness that occurred when a drop of it got on my face horrified me. Several hours later the burning and redness turned raw. That quarter sized raw sore spot from adulterated oil lasted for weeks... *on my face!* Every time I looked in the mirror I was reminded of how dangerous adulterated oils could be.

Another experience that cemented my loyalty to Young Living Essential Oils again occurred in my early training. I used several oils that were labeled "pure and natural" from an unknown company that the distributor was insisting were therapeutic grade. My results were an unpleasant buzzing sensation everywhere I had put this oil. My fingertips which I used to apply the oil "buzzed" for several days.

I learned my lesson the hard way about using inferior oils. Learn from my pain, okay? Now that I have fully clarified that you must know and trust your Essential Oil provider, please choose wisely. Understand clearly that marketing terms, unscientific testing, and bad information is bountiful and could be dangerous if you aren't careful.

Please do not use inferior oils. You are not an inferior person. You deserve the best of God's world, demand this from those that create the crap world. Do not buy their poisons! Without your support, they will either come around or go away. It's all driven by greed and perpetuated by lack of awareness on the part of the consumer. Awareness is our best defense.

Raindrops Save the Day

The following are my experiences and results with Therapeutic Grade Essential Oils in regards to managing pain and other symptoms in daily life as a chemical sensitive and chemical intolerant individual. I believe their daily usage has helped me prevent further liver troubles. Therapeutic Grade Essential Oils are a vast subject worthy of your study. I find that after nineteen years of intensive usage and study there is always more to learn and share. For more information on purchasing books on the subject of Essential Oils, see Resources section in the back of this book.

My next significant experience with using therapeutic grade Essential Oils came after a year of using peppermint oil for pain relief. I had started to experiment with more and more Young Living Essential Oils. I was intrigued by Heather's book on Essential Oils called *Essential Oils Desk Reference (2nd Edition)* and it contained a section called **Raindrop Technique®** which involved using several oils at once.

After experiencing what just a single drop had been able to thwart, I was very interested in what several drops of oils could do... painous interuptus, ahhhhh! Relief! I was eager for more pain relief! Being chemical intolerant often means painful days and nights.

I was seeking pain relief from chronic neck pain from a decades old injury. When I was 16 years old I had fallen on my head and compressed my neck in a gymnastic tumbling accident. This injury left me with a neck that was often stiff, painful, and always with limited mobility. In fact I could not fully look over my left shoulder. I often spent great amounts of money on the chiropractor for adjustments, as my neck would on occasion just seize up leaving me helpless and in pain for days. I was not even considering what a Raindrop Technique® session would or could do for my old neck injury *per se*. I was motivated to try Raindrop Technique® for relief from chronic pain *due* to the old neck injury.

During my first Raindrop Technique® session my back turned very red except for a big white spot over my left lung area. (I had pneumonia in my left lung as a child). Although my skin was very red, it didn't hurt. In fact it felt great, warm and entrenching is more how I would describe the sensations. When my session was completed I put my arms under my body to lift myself up into a sitting position. That's when I heard a "pop", and then the sound of falling dominoes in my head. And in that moment my neck suddenly released! The sounds were audible enough that Heather and the other woman in the room looked shocked and worried. The noise sounded like a broken neck! But it wasn't. From that day on I could look **fully** over my left shoulder.

This therapeutic technique was developed by Gary Young founder of Young Living Essential Oils (YLEO), after he observed the elders of the Lakota tribe perform healings on tribal members. This technique has been shown to reduce microbe activity within the spine. For over fifteen years I have used this effective and safe therapeutic technique on a regular basis with only positive beneficial results. It's a large part of my regiment for preventive care and my reward was that it gave me back my immune system.

Each week I could feel the effects as the powerful oils cleared pathogens out of my injured tissues, encouraged the detoxing of my cells from petrochemicals, and supported my spiritual, mental and emotional bodies. I stopped being overcome by sudden opportunistic infections and chronic pain was lessening. After the big chemical exposure in 2005 a Raindrop Technique® session would purge copious amounts of mucus from my body, leaving me able to breath and feeling lighter with each session.

It would take another ten years of regular Raindrop Technique® sessions before the big white spot on my back finally filled in with red. Each session would break up more of that scar tissue within my lung and my breathing became deeper and fuller. Cold weather no longer "took my breath away" and I found that I didn't get so winded after physical exertion.

In my humble opinion Raindrop Technique® is just the perfect medicine: it's preventive, proactive, restorative, and beneficial for both receiver and giver, and anyone else in the area of the fragrance!

Raindrop Technique® is easy to learn. You can find a buddy, buy A Raindrop Technique® Essential Oil Collection from Young Living and learn to do it for yourselves. I know you will be happy you did. If you don't want to learn it, then I encourage you to seek out a Raindrop Technique® practitioner certified by Center for Aromatherapy Research and Education (CARE).

"Since the potential benefits of Raindrop Technique depend on the quality of the oils applied requires that CCIs (Certified Care

Instructor student) use only Young Living oils when practicing or teaching in the name of CARE. If other brands of verifiable therapeutic grade oils become available, that requirement may be modified in the future. CARE training programs are open to everyone..."

From The Center For Aromatherapy Research Website
www.raindroptraining.com/care/yleo.shtml

There are high end spas that offer Raindrop Technique® at $250 or more a session. A Raindrop Technique® Essential Oil Collection is more budget friendly and can provide you with several sessions. Ordering information to purchase your own **The Raindrop Technique® Essential Oil Collection** will be found in Resources. You will get 5 ml bottles of each oil necessary to do Raindrop Technique® which is enough to do at least 8 raindrop sessions if not more. You can then slowly add in the 15 ml bottles and for that size you can do many more raindrop sessions.

How to Begin a Relationship with God's Medicine

It's advisable that one begin with using the oils externally first before ingesting them. Taking time and experiencing these wonderful oils allows your body the experience of the healing power of each oil. With each new oil you experience, begin with an inhalation of the oil. Open the bottle of oil and hold it down low below your nose (at waist level), slowly bring the oil up, towards your nose, allowing the different compounds to float up towards your nostrils. Take notice of how your body reacts. Keeping a slow pace and gently bringing the oil up slowly to your nose, allowing the Essential Oil to enter your body via the nasal passages and into your limbic system, the emotional center of your brain, the hub of your emotions.

The easiest and safest place to apply any new Essential Oil is to the bottom of the feet. This allows the body time to acquaint itself with this healing support from God's intended medicine, the plant. Another way to get acquainted is to put oils on the belly around the navel area.

The two Essential Oils that I avoid even with Young Living Essential Oils are neroli and jasmine they must be extracted with solvents. (in this book neroli and jasmine in blends are marked with a ^) Although these solvent are technically removed in the distillation process, for me as a chemical intolerant individual I avoid the use of these two Essential Oils as singles. However jasmine is in blends I like to use and I have had good results. Just be aware. I know about the solvent distraction method because Young Living informed me. Again its very important to know your supplier of Essential Oils and how the plant is processed from the seed, soil and all the way through to the distillation process.

Once I felt comfortable with how my body reacted with these therapeutic oils, I took it to the next level by ingesting the ones labeled as "Supplement." When I feel the threat of illness, I grab my oils and I take them internally for several days until I feel I'm securely back in homeostasis. My use of therapeutic Essential Oils has been my "go to medication" for over nineteen years! It has shown me the power of the body to heal with plant medicine.

Dilution with a high grade fatty oil like sesame oil or almond oil is desirable. This helps stop any burning sensation the Essential Oil may have. Oregano is an Essential Oil that can feel like it's burning the skin, it's an irritant and is advisable to use a high quality carrier oil with this especially with young children.

Note for Children: <u>Children under age three should have oils diluted with a carrier oil.</u> Some oils are irritating on tender young skin and dilution is more comfortable. It's not necessary to be uncomfortable with therapeutic grade Essential Oils. I find it's preferable to dilute Essential Oils fifty fifty (one drop of carrier oil to one drop of Essential Oil) in a carrier oil for little kids and apply to the bottom of their feet. I use Young Living's V-6 oil, its light, convenient and a little goes a long way.

Improving the Inner Environment

Another way I benefit from therapeutic grade Essential Oils is to take them internally. This practice has been of great benefit to my survival and my relief from petroleum and heavy metal poisoning. Before I get into taking therapeutic grade Essential Oils internally, I want to make two more important points on the subject.

First point is about how our government in the United States looks at labeling. If the product is a food it will have a "Nutritional" label. If the product isn't a food, but is a supplement to nutrition then it has a label for "Supplement" and is for ingesting. FDA regulations also state a product cannot be labeled for use as a dietary supplement AND for topical or aromatic use, both can not be on the same label.

Many of the Young Living Oils have a supplement label and all their labels have directions, however to be in full compliance with the FDA regulations Young Living has recently begun displaying labels that distinguish the products intended as a dietary supplement and those intended to be used for topical application or aromatic use. Young Living's new labels are on the Vitality line of therapeutic grade essential oils. These are the same 100% therapeutic-grade essential oils for which Young Living has become known, with a new label. The Vitality line has been created so you can now draw clear distinction between topical/aromatic use and dietary use. This should drastically reduce any confusion!

Further clarification from Young Living states: *"The ingredients in our Dietary supplements and foods are approved by the FDA for consumption. The ingredients in our cosmetics are approved by the FDA for cosmetic use. The FDA has not approved Young Living's products but the ingredients used in our products.*

Young Living has a Claims Committee reviewing all current scientific research to determine the label for each product. Federal regulations require sufficient scientific evidence to support the label of the product. This means that any Young Living® product will require sufficient evidence to determine usage and following the usage directions will help ensure the safety and efficacy of the product."

In 2007 the FDA issued a Good Manufacturing Practices (GMPs) for dietary supplements. This is a set of requirements and expectations by which dietary supplements must be manufactured, prepared, and stored to ensure quality. That leaves the therapeutic value up to the manufacturer to determine through additional voluntary channels and certification processes. From my experience its important to trust that your Essential Oil supplier is practicing Good Manufacturing Practices and not illusionary marketing tactics.

The second and last important note to make before anyone with or without multiple chemical sensitivities or chemical intolerance starts ingesting Essential Oils needs to be aware of are potential detoxing results. Over the years, a side effect of using therapeutic grade essentials oils as my medicine was an increase in cleansing reactions from the detox of petroleum chemicals. Yes, it sometimes is a challenge to go through the detox period; but getting to the other side of being sick and polluted with petrochemicals was well worth the effort to get through it!

Therapeutic grade Essential Oils are my medicine and they've been essential in helping me help return myself back to homeostasis. Eventually therapeutic grade Essential Oils became an everyday tool for me. I continue to use them for supporting my body to remain in homeostasis and protecting me from petroleum based chemicals down on a molecular level.

Ideas for Ingesting Essential Oils:

- Start with one drop. Essential Oils can be up to 100 times stronger than their dried herb counter part.

- Add a drop or two to a smoothie.

- Put the desired drops into a veggie capsule, take promptly.

- Prepare food with them, adding them into your dish at the end of cooking/heating, <u>High prolonged heat destroys the therapeutic value of Essential Oils.</u>

- Put desired drops into a fat/oil based, non-polluted substance such as organic olive oil, almond milk, or my favorite... coconut milk. Honey will also work. You can use a small glass or a spoon.

- **Note:** Plastic and Essential Oils do not mix! Do not use plastic spoons or cups. Do not put Essential Oils into plastic water bottles. Vessels made of glass are best. A dedicated shot glass works well. I use a small two ounce glass. Whichever you choose to use, fill it half full with your milk and then add your desired therapeutic grade Essential Oil drops. If you use a spoon you can stir your milk and Essential Oil with a toothpick if you want but that takes coordination. I just swallow mine down without another to do about it. If you get some on your lips and it burns, just rub oil on it to cool the burning sensation. Real organic soft butter or coconut oil will work also, as well as a dab of milk will soothe it... you get the idea? It's not hard and it's not scary. All you need to remember is what? Use 100% Therapeutic Grade Essential Oils Within You and Upon You.

Improving the Outer Environment

Essential Oils and:
- **Multiple Chemical Sensitivity**
- **Chemical Intolerance**
- **Environmental Illness**
- **Idiopathic Environmental Intolerance**

You may be wondering what does all this have to do with MCS, CI, EI, and IEI besides to be aware of the synthetic, adulterated Essential Oils? Therapeutic Essential Oils are one of the missing links between your body and true healing support, it's one of the simplest and easiest things you can do for yourself. It's one of the best ways I found to escape the chemical world of pharmaceuticals.

These type of oils are a gift from God and designed by nature to be our true medicine. Therapeutic grade Essential Oils are the leaves in the biblical directive "use the leaves of the river for your medicine." The bible didn't say "bring up the black crude oil from beneath the earth, boil it and let it be your medicine."

There was no plan in the bible for our environment to become an atmosphere of benzene.

In an atmosphere of benzene the best method of application is to diffuse the oils, for this you will need to purchase a cold air diffuser (see Resources). Diffusing helps the MCS, CI, EI, and IEI sufferer tolerate the intolerable environments. Diffusing is when a few drops of therapeutic grade Essential Oil is dispensed via a boost of cool air, splitting the Essential Oil drop into a million micro bursts of oil droplets, out and into the environment. Diffusing some Essential Oils can disinfectant the air without harmful petrochemicals, creating a safer environment.[4]

Essential Oils used in the home to clean and disinfect on a daily basis deter insects. Most oils can be diffused, however some are too thick and others can be irritating if diffused too long. Young Living has directions for use on each bottle, for special diffusing times.

As a Chemical Intolerant survivor, I use therapeutic grade Essential Oils on my body. This helps me tolerate certain environments that are notorious danger zones for petrochemical exposure such as gas stations, airplanes, and hospitals. I keep Frankincense oil on me at all times to protect me from sneak petrochemical environmental exposure. In the past, I would diffuse

Essential Oils at work to help with the constant threat of chemicals in the environment. It was amusing to observe how co-workers always seemed to make their way over to my work space with an excuse to come smell my air.

For those with Environmental Illness, therapeutic grade Essential Oils help calm down the over inflamed nervous system. Diffusing oils helps to gently calm down the fire of the exhausted nervous system with oils such as lavender, patchouli, valerian, rose, and the Young Living blend labeled "Peace and Calming." There are many oils to try, but these are the specific ones that helped me when my system was over taxed from the environment.

How Does It Help?

#1) Enhances healing of mental, emotional, and spiritual: When you breath in the molecules of a therapeutic grade Essential Oil (or the molecules of anything else for that matter) these molecules go immediately up the nostrils and onto the olfactory bulbs and on into the limbic area of the brain. The limbic area of the brain is the portion of the brain that deals with emotions, memories and stimulation as well as connects to other deeper parts of the brain.

#2) Enhances healing of physical on the cellular level: Therapeutic grade Essential Oils help the individual by working within the cells of our body's, by gently penetrating the cell wall and can enter through the blood brain barrier. There are some therapeutic grade Essential Oils that are able to purge pathogens from our cells. Other therapeutic Essential Oils dissolve petroleum from receptor sites. All therapeutic Essential Oils have proven to increase blood flow, delivering oxygen and nutrients to each cell. These are a few of the many exciting happenings in your molecules when Essential Oils join the party!

#3) Antimicrobial and Detoxifying: The antimicrobial effects of Essential Oils have been well researched and published in many peer reviewed journals such as the Oxford Journal, as well as papers and abstracts presented by researchers for the food and pharmaceutical industry. These Essential Oil studies support the effectiveness of Essential Oils on antimicrobial activities. These studies are conducted by researchers from around the world with much of this research taking place outside of the United States, with the exception of a few; Weber University in Ogden, Utah, The Smell and Taste Research Foundation in Chicago, Illinois, and the H. Lee Moffitt Cancer Center, Tampa Florida.

The National Institute of Health has posted a study on the antimicrobial effects of several therapeutic grade Essential Oils such as clove, oregano, and cinnamon. A 1999 study of 52 plant oils by the Department of Microbiology at the University of Western Australia,[5] found twenty of these essential oils to have inhibitory actions on eleven microbes including *Candida albicans* and *Staphylococcus aureus* (the MRSA strain of bacteria). You can read the entire abstract here:
http://www.ncbi.nlm.nih.gov/pubmed/?term=10438227

In my not so distant past one of my entertainment industry jobs was located in a moldy building. Management was not cooperating with me on how best to cleanse the moldy dank environment. They wanted me to use chlorine bleach and another industrial chemical, and I wanted to use aromatherapy. As we discussed the severity of the situation from my point of view, the janitor turned on a water vacuum to complete cleaning up the overwhelming wet mess making the mold. Within seconds the invisible bacteria and mold spores blowing thru the air over took me. I was wracked with sneezing spasms so rapid fire I had to quickly exit the building. The frustrated look on my supervisor's face revealed that he had not believed me when in my initial interview I had revealed my confirmed medical diagnosis of my allergy to toluene aka methyl benzene, dust and mold. For the first and only time in my career aromatherapy and the use of Essential Oils was approved for in the costume budget.

I personally have experienced pain, infection, injury and chemical intolerance symptoms improve with the use of these wonderful oils. Daily use can happen in several ways, by direct application, diffusing, and ingesting. With daily use of the oils, and regular Raindrop Technique sessions, getting the flu and flu like symptoms and colds are no longer my main activity. My allergies are easier to manage. I continue to have many wonderful experiences with these oils.

However, the best experience for me as a Chemical Intolerant individual was the experience of Frankincense and how it has allowed me to move about this petroleum based society with less impact and devastation upon my personal health and well being.

The Gift of Kings

One day after listening to a few lectures on the power of Frankincense I decided to take this oil internally. The research I found was supporting Frankincense as an Essential Oil that changed the spin of the pineal gland. The pineal gland is located in the brain and some people refer to it as the "third eye." It's role in our health is very important, as it's one of the master glands that rules over homeostasis. The pineal is the part of the brain most benefited from the ancient practice of "stillness within" and is why meditation benefits our health and well being.

In one of the lectures was a simple statement of how the Frankincense molecule would bind itself to the petrochemical molecular "goo" stuck in the cellular receptor sites, thus helping support the cell's excretion of this toxic "goo." I was excited by this piece of news! It gave me the justification in my mind to be extravagant as Frankincense was in the luxury price range of my budget for an Essential Oil. It would turn out that it was a bargain for what it would do for supporting my well being.

For ten months, starting in August of 2002 all the way until May of 2003, I took three to five drops of Frankincense internally one to two times a day. My results were unexpected and changed my idea of what was possible with therapeutic grade Essential Oils.

Within days of starting the Frankincense the chronic pain in my right elbow abruptly stopped. At about three months into taking the Frankincense internally I noticed my mind was calmer and my immune system was staying strong. While my co workers came down with the usual colds and flu, I remained healthy. These side effects along with the abrupt relief from my elbow's chronic pain gave me the confidence to stay with my Frankincense experience. Six months of ingesting the therapeutic grade Frankincense, marked the beginning of a memorable transformation of my delicate, weak, and frail right elbow, a transformation that went beyond my wildest dreams.

My right elbow's downward descent began decades ago. In my early twenties with a bad fall resulting in a medical diagnosis of a minor and inconvenient muscle injury and bone bruise. At that time I had the habit of rubbing a well know well established pain relief creme on the area. When I was a kid this product gave me great relief, but like the aspirin in the mid seventies, one day treating this elbow injury the creme gave me a rash. (This injury happened right before my toluene allergy was confirmed). In 1980 full relief never came for my painful injured elbow. From thereafter that elbow was tender, sore, and troubled by pain and weakness until I started the Frankincense regime. Understand that for the pain and soreness of decades to abruptly stop within days of starting the Frankincense regime, it grabbed my attention.

A few more weeks into the Frankincense treatment the elbow became hot to the touch, and had red streaks and swirls around the area. Each day there was a different pattern to the red streaks. One day looking in the mirror I realized that's what my elbow had looked like all those years ago when I used the white pain relief creme, only this was in reverse.

In the past the streaks would be white with medication waiting to soak in, whereas today it was red with inflammation. I felt it best to continue to trust the Frankincense and the detox process. After all, the pain of many years had abruptly stopped, and although the area was hot, delightfully I was not in pain. Eventually after several more weeks the redness turned into cracked skin that flaked away ("dermatitis" according to one doctor). Each day that passed, that elbow became stronger and once again flexible with soft, smooth skin. This experience took about ten months from ingesting the first drop of Frankincense to the complete healing of smooth new beautiful skin, and the pain in that elbow never returned!

This taught me a valuable lesson in how the body stores petrochemicals and releases them with Frankincense. I watched and felt the release of petrochemical molecules exiting my elbow without fear or trepidation. I trusted the process. It lead me to an understanding that it was stored benzene molecules leaving my elbow. My experience of observing the process of detoxification uninterrupted to completion was up close and personal.

Most Frankincense comes from Somalia, however there is another type of Frankincense grown only in Oman. This one is called Sacred Frankincense and is very beneficial for skin, lymph, and cancer issues. I have noticed this Sacred Frankincense coupled with Essential Oil of Ocotea diminishes the stress from amoeba, as well.

From that time onward I use either of these varieties of Frankincense on me before I leave the house or if I 'm going to be meeting a new person. I put at least one drop a day under my nose or on my temples. This is my invisible "mask of protection" and it's another way I'm able to stay alive and well in a society saturated in benzene.

Maximum Healing with Synthesis

The blends are when two or more oils have been mixed together creating a synergistic formulation of oils, giving the maximum benefit for a specific intent. I choose formulation blends from Young Living Essential Oils that contain Frankincense with other therapeutic grade Essential Oils. Choosing your oils this way may give you maximum benefit as you begin your journey. Below are some blends that I've used to help me in my journey back to health.

Believe™ - I would use this in meditation and prayer, increasing the belief that I could become well and strong again. I apply under my nose and affirm the belief that I am normal, and it's the benzene that does not belong. It is good to diffuse this blend.

Brain Power™ - This powerful blend was created by Gary Young, the founder of Young Living Therapeutic Essential Oils, with the intention to help remove the petrochemicals coating the brain. Once this coating is removed mental focus increases and relieves the "brain fog" that petroleum based chemicals create in the brain. I like to use this blend with peppermint anytime I feel a slight headache approaching and using the peppermint rushes it away.

Transformation™ - Diffuse this blend of Frankincense, Idaho Balsam Fir, Rosemary, and Cardamon helps remove the imprint of negative emotions from our cells and bring us into a new mindset. Diffuse this blend for best results.

Trauma Life™ - The name says it all. Petrochemicals create trauma on the cells and organs, as well as the emotional and mental trauma that comes from being a sick, chemical sensitive citizen in a benzene nation.

Valor™ - This blend contains Frankincense with blue tansy, spruce, rosewood designed by Dr. Young to help one face the day with courage and confidence.

White Angelica™ - This blend is formulated with high frequency oils such as Rose, Sandalwood and Myrrh. These higher vibration oils clear negativity from the environment and strengthen the aura. This blend has helped me calm down when energy from the environment was overwhelming me. The fragrance is lovely and subtly helps others release negativity when in the presence of it's aroma.

Supporting the Immune System

The USDA researchers at Tufts University in Boston, have a test that is able to measure the antioxidant capacity of food. This test is called the ORAC an acronym for Oxygen Radical Absorbance Capacity. ORAC measures both time and degree of free radical inhibition of a food. Benzene, chlorine, and mold create free radical damage, so inhibiting them is part of staying well. Before I knew and understood the ORAC scale, any exposure to benzene or chlorine and my immune system would take a dive. Back in the days before I had my solutions, I would have a sore throat in minutes, an earache in hours, flu like symptoms and bedridden for days. I learned to use the ORAC as a score card for which foods would best support my immune system.

Clove - Clove oil has been used throughout the ages to help ward off plagues and pestilence. This single Essential Oil is the least expensive but will give me the biggest relief anytime my immune system needs help. On the ORAC scale Clove oil scores the highest! Clove comes in over a half million above other Essential Oils and over one million higher than foods in antioxidant absorption on the ORAC scale. When I put a drop of this oil on the bottom of each foot I know I'm supporting my immune system. Clove oil has protected my immune system when others around me were succumbing to the flu. It's another oil I always have on hand. One day as I was looking at the bottle of clove oil it jumped out at me "With clove you "c" love" It stuck me as funny but true. Clove is a true wonder Essential Oil and I "c" love as often as I can!

Exodus II™ - This blend contains Frankincense with other powerful therapeutic grade Essential Oils that contain germ killing compounds and in turn are supportive to the immune system.

Hope™ - This blend is formulated with **Melissa** oil, a potent antiviral and immune stimulant.

A Healthy Mouth Without Chemicals

My mouth is often one of the first organs of my digestive system to let me know we've been invaded by chemicals. My gums were an early casualty of my chemical sensitivities. Many toothpaste are saturated with petrochemicals and this would keep my mouth full of irritations that were becoming more bothersome. Seeking out non chemical containing mouth care often left me with baking soda and peroxide as my best options. Thankfully there are more choices available as more and more consumers become aware of the dangers of absorbing benzene and fluoride in the delicate sublingual areas of the mouth.

My family loves to use tooth pastes containing Essential Oils and no benzene or fluoride. I have listed them in the Resources. The Essential Oils within the toothpaste support my gums health that I rarely have gum pain and oral health problems any more, but when I did these are some of my solutions:

Oregano - It's important to <u>dilute oregano</u> by using equal drops of a carrier oil. Oregano is a powerful bactericide and is excellent for stopping clostridium, a nasty bacteria in the mouth. Hulda Clark,[6] a cancer researcher, writer and truth seeker regarding toxicity and pathogens and their role in cancer, found dissected cancer tumors to have clostridium bacteria in the center of the mass (along with heavy metals and other undesirables). <u>Oregano can irritate the skin</u> and mouth, be sure to <u>dilute with a carrier oil</u> until experience is gained with this Essential Oil. Oregano was worth the effort to master using correctly, it's an amazing healing oil for dental troubles. Oregano oil is strong, but not as harmful as it feels, I actually accidentally got some in my eye and was expecting the worse pain, but after three minutes it was fine, however lips are irritated by it. Dilution is suggested. Before I use it on my toothbrush I rub coconut oil on my lips to protect them from irritation from the Oregano oil. Another way is to mix a few drops of oregano to a tablespoon of baking soda mix together and brush.

Clove - I put a drop on my toothbrush with chemical free toothpaste when I feel my gums are in trouble. I have also used clove to stop an aching tooth. It helps rid my mouth of bad breath.

Peppermint - A drop in my mouth takes care of most of my tooth troubles, bad breath, stomachaches, and headaches. It also can be added to a toothbrush for a truly refreshing experience.

Ocotea - This is a plant of the Rainforest. I take this oil internally to keep microbes like amoeba under control in my gums as well as in my lymph system.

Support for Hormones

To be honest, I had an easier time with menopause than I did with menstruation and PMS. Now I know why. It was the petroleum chemicals clogging up my receptor sites! Once the receptor site is full of goo, the hormones cannot make their connection, enzymes are not delivered properly to the hormone receptor sites, and hormones go out of whack. There is great relief for the body when the receptor sites are cleared of goo and the hormones and enzyme activity within the body can come into balance and homeostasis returns as the true normal.

There are several ways to use the oils for this purpose:

- Diffuse
- Inhale
- Directly place on bottom of feet.
- Use hot compress.
- Dilute in massage oil for body massage.

Therapeutic essential single oils that are supportive for both PMS and menopause are:

- **Clary Sage**
- **Sage**
- **Frankincense**
- **Lavender**

Therapeutic essential single oils that are supportive for men and promote male hormone and prostrate balancing:

- **Blue Cypress**
- **Cedarwood**
- **Fennel**
- **Frankincense**
- **Geranium**
- **Rosemary**

The main therapeutic blends from Young Living Essential Oils that support hormones; (marked with a ^ contains neroli and/or jasmine)

For Women:

- **Lady Sclareol**™^
- **Dragontime**™^
- **Joy**™^
- **Ylang-Ylang**
- **Peace and Calming**™,
- **SARA**™

For Men:

- **Endoflex**™
- **Mister**™

The Rebellious Belly

Peppermint - I cannot share enough the wonderment of Peppermint for stomach relief. Rub it on the navel or take a drop internally. It stops my stomach from rebellion tactics. Peppermint is also known to help your stomach realize its full by stimulating receptors in the brain to shut off your appetite. It has helped me calm down a sugar binge attack as well as stop bad breath.

Clove - Is another single oil that when I ingested a few drops has given me relief from bloating and gas. I have had very good results with taking clove internally when I suspected food poisoning.

In the oil blends of Young Living Essential Oils there are several that have helped me with tummy troubles. These oil blends rubbed on my navel area at bedtime has helped me get a stuck bowel to release.

- **Release**™
- **Juva Flex**™
- **Di Gize**™

Managing Pain and Fever

Essential Oil usage has helped me to make the leap from victim to victor over pain and fevers. I can now live a fuller life and manage pain, never resorting to over the counter petrochemical medications. Out of all the single oils I've used to grant relief from pain the top three winners are **Peppermint**, **Clove**, and **Lemongrass** and the best blend from Young Living is **Panaway**.

Panaway™ - Is a Young Living Essential Oil blend formulated with Essential Oils of helichrysum and peppermint is known for their pain stopping abilities. It works wonders and is great to have in your home's Essential Oil first aid kit. Apply directly on the painful areas. This oil blend can also be applied to the bottom of feet for small children. For broken skin apply to the bottom feet or navel area.

Note for Children: Children under three should have oils diluted with a carrier oil at a ratio of one to one. Some oils are irritating on tender, young skin and dilution is more comfortable. It's not necessary to be temporarily uncomfortable with therapeutic grade Essential Oils. As I mentioned earlier you can use Young Living's V-6 oil for diluting. It's light, convenient, and a little goes a long way. However, organic coconut oil and other organic oils like olive or sesame can also be used. Please use only organic, or it will be counter productive. **Do not put peppermint oil on the neck of children under age three, and always use carrier oils to dilute 50:50 or one on one when placing oils on children under the age of three.** When in doubt the safest place to apply oils on anyone is the bottom of the feet.

Peppermint - For myself for a fever a drop of peppermint on the bottom of my feet, drop a few drops onto my spine and gently rub around. Then I wrap up in warm blankets, as peppermint cools the body down so fast that it can feel like a chill. I love a hot towel or heating pad over my feet when this happens. Peppermint oil has potent capabilities to overcome harmful bacteria.

Lavender - A few drops of lavender on a cold compress have also brought me relief when I was simply overheated, which is easy to do in the tropics. I found for a child that it helps calm them down when they have a fever. Putting a drop of diluted peppermint oil on the bottom of their feet is fun and comforting when followed by lavender.

Lemongrass – Besides helping lift the mood in the environment Lemongrass is very helpful for tendon and other connective tissue pain. Lemongrass is also good for fighting fungus as well.

I found the help and support my body needed from therapeutic Essential Oils. I have nineteen years of personal experience through usage and observation, as well as many hours listening to and reading through research complied on Essential Oils. I have read several editions of the *Essential Oils Desk Reference (first edition through fifth edition)* from Life Science Publishing (see Resources for most recent editions) as well as Gary Young's *Essential Oils Integrative Medical Guide.* After all this time I've yet to find another therapeutic grade Essential Oil company that has the science, the research, and personal experience that I found with the Young Living Essential Oils (YLEO) company. That's why at this time they're the only

Essential Oil company I can recommend.

Young Living Essential Oils is a company working to ensure confidence in purity and the highest of effectiveness in therapeutic results from a complete 100% pure therapeutic grade Essential Oil born from the leaves of the valley.

Essential Oils are our lifeline back to what medicine was meant to be. Medicine was always intended to be from the leaves of the river and teaming with life; not made from the dead things of another eon, buried deep in the crude.

<u>Chapter Ten</u>

The Professor and A New Science

*"The state of mind which enables a man to do work of this kind...
is akin to that of the religious worshiper or the lover; the daily
effort comes from no deliberate intention or program, but straight
from the heart."*
~Albert Einstein~

The second solution for my chemical intolerance came into my life after almost dying from that last big chemical exposure during the preparation of the *Miami Vice* feature film. I was very sick and as I described earlier in Chapter 8, I didn't bounce back quickly. My health had been permanently and negatively affected. I had no energy and could barely drag myself out of bed, let alone go to work. My usual solution of Essential Oil usage needed back up.

After this catastrophic exposure my awareness of chemicals was dramatically heightened, which I didn't think was possible. I could smell every cigarette within 50 feet, and the exhaust from generators and cars nauseated me. Each morning people's deodorant and after shave became menacing odor bombs out to kill me. After a trip through the production office or the crew work areas I was weak and winded because this is where perfume, microwave popcorn fumes, permanent markers, paint, special effects, hair, and make up created chemical clouds of devastation for me.

The symptoms I displayed were intense and varied. My skin had a funny, dull look to it. My hair was lackluster. My eyes were tearing and so red and painful that I wore my sunglasses indoors. My feet swelled and felt like they were on fire!

Most food upset my stomach and caused me to be constipated so I couldn't eat much and yet all of my clothes were too tight. I was swelling fast. I ordered a week's worth of work clothes in a larger size and when they arrived they were already too tight.

Every time I bent over I wanted to cry because my head throbbed from the pressure and pain of impacted mucus and my skull was so heavy I felt like I would fall over from the weight of it. At night my sleep was interrupted with night sweats and multiple trips to the bathroom.

I needed help. I needed something different. Doctors couldn't help me and medicine would certainly kill me. I needed to find Valentina, the lady in red, along with the bio-resonance device that helped my son. Bio-resonance technology had proven to be one of the few options available for someone with any chemical issues.

The search for Valentina lead me to an updated Bio-resonance device that was similar to hers, but later I would learn this new device was far more advanced. My friend Heather met a woman who owned and operated this new device. Unfortunately, Heather could not locate the women and she only remembered that the name of the device included the letters "QX."

When I googled QX and that's when the face of angel popped up. My internet searches led me to find Professor William Nelson and the device that would soon change my life: his "QX" energetic medical device. Which I came to learn is actually the first letters of the first device developed, a QXCI and the latest device to buy in 2005 was a SCIO. Today in 2016 the most updated device is the EDUCTOR. The EDUCTOR carries a Platinum rating from the World Health Products Ratings Service. The EDUCTOR is the world's most validated and legally registered device to date. (See Resources)

In order to understand what this equipment is and how it works, it's important to know some of Professor Nelson's history. The following information is adapted from Professor Nelson's official biography from the book *Angel Messenger* written by Desire Dubounet. (See Resources)

Professor Nelson is an American math genius who at age 15 attained a perfect I.Q. score and he was accepted into MENSA at age 16. At 19 years old, Nelson was chosen out of 15,000 college math student applicants for General Motors Institute in the math department to work on their space projects during Apollo missions 11, 12, and 13. In order to arrive alive, Apollo 13 needed navigational coordinates to safely hit their intended target (a boat) in a vast ocean. This young math genius, working behind the scenes, calculated the correct mathematical solution that would ultimately bring Apollo 13 within 150 meters of it's intended pick up target.

He is also deeply spiritual. As a youth he studied the Bible in Greek, Hebrew, Latin, and English. Ultimately Bill Nelson chose to attend seminary and become a pastor. During his studies at seminary his teachers explained that God calls each of the students to service, and they would often ask, "Did you get the calling?" When Bill received his calling from God it came with instructions to re-write molecular biology. It seemed important to young Nelson to learn all about molecular biology if he was going to re-write it. He earned his bachelor of science in Psychology and his masters of science in Counseling Psychology at Youngstown. He also studied Biology at the University of Wisconsin and Quantum Physics at Kent State.

A result of his college studies was young Nelson's epiphany that quantum theory could better explain the biological principals for molecular biology than the current science of thermodynamics. In 1982 Professor Nelson published these concepts in his first book, *The Promorpheus*.[1] The title Promorpheus refers to the first shape of biology as we know it. Promorpheus is derived from the word promorphology. Promorphology is a branch of bio science; the scientific study of living organisms. Promorphology is the branch of bio science that studies the forms of organisms from a mathematical point of view.[2]

Since 1982, Professor Nelson has written over one hundred books, written and produced over fifty multimedia productions, plus published over eighty papers on brain physiology, NLP[3] (neuro- linguistic programming), mathematics, reactivity, electroceuticals,[4] and the powers of the mind. He's a mathematician, researcher, developer, medical lecturer, (and in my opinion) hero, who has turned his intelligence to finding a natural cure for cancer.

However, what is most important to you and I, is that Professor Nelson has written numerous books on the proof that synthetic food and drugs are not compatible with the human body. Nelson's approach brings a new solution to the many challenges one may face when carrying a toxic overload. This new science has helped me recover and I believe it can help all those suffering with Multiple Chemical Sensitivity (MCS), Chemical Intolerance (CI), Environmental Illness (EI), and Idiopathic Environmental Intolerance (IEI).

As part of my continued research, I watched every YouTube video on "QX", "Professor William Nelson", or anything on the subject of quantum physics and healing. In the videos Professor Nelson laid out ideas that were new for me. New ideas with new terms like "Nelsonian Medicine", "voltammetric", "exhaustion phase", "Body Electric" and "the SUPERconscious mind". (In the next section I will define these important terms.) With this new information, I felt clarity. I totally got Nelsonian medicine. For the first time in a long time I found a form of medicine that could involve me!

Tomorrow's Medicine Today

It was easy to see I needed to get one of Professor Nelson's devices in order to stay alive. I was determined to get well. In addition to my chronic lack of funds, it turned out my options for purchasing were also limited. Since I wasn't a licensed health care provider, the brokers wouldn't sell me a device.

Eventually I found a broker who would sell me the device, along with a student package he offered that included three days of training with Professor Nelson, plus financing. Additionally, the president of the brokerage required me to participate in a device demonstration prior to purchase. Traveling to the demonstration, my poor health turned a six hour, round trip drive into a twelve hour excursion across The Florida Everglades and back. The entire experience was complicated because a major hurricane had left my region highly disorganized and in the dark. However, I knew I needed to purchase the device. I was determined to get to that demonstration even if it meant crossing The Everglades alone, sick, without street lights, road signs, rest stops, and limited access to gasoline.

Once I arrived the practitioner started the demonstration immediately. This particular practitioner was using the SCIO, which stands for Scientific Consciousness Interface Operations System and is just one of the devices developed by Nelson. The practitioner placed rubber straps on my head, wrists and ankles. These rubber feeling straps were actual electrodes made of graphite and are used to detect the subtle skin changes that take place with stress. I then sat in an easy chair with my feet up on an ottoman. The practitioner began to ask me questions. First it was basic information like my name, birthday, and the time and place of my birth. Then she began to ask me unusual questions about my daily habits, past injuries, and traumas. I was to answer on a one to ten scale, with zero or one being little to no stress and ten being the worst stress.

After a few minutes of this simple dialogue she told me to sit quietly as she "calibrated" the device to me. I felt gentle waves of relaxing energy and wondered if that was the treatment. Before I could ask, she told me we were going to the next step, which is to run the galvanized skin response. This would identify what stress I was reacting to so that the device could then run the needed "retraining" programs to help my body better handle the effects of stress. (I would later learn that "retraining" is a term to replace the medical word "therapy.")

Thirty minutes into the session the mucus pressure pain in my head stopped throbbing. After forty five minutes I could take a deep breath. It was the first deep breath I had taken in five months that didn't end in a coughing spasm. All the tightness in my chest relaxed. My vision seemed a little clearer and my mind felt tuned up. After an hour I began to feel hopeful for the future! My results were so amazing that with complete confidence I took a giant step into the world of quantum healing; right then and there I pulled out my credit card and completed the purchase.

This town's local grocery store had their electricity back on and were re-stocked. I actually felt well enough to go shopping (something I'd been unable to do for months). That night, with bags of groceries beside me, I joyfully drove back across The Everglades in the smothering darkness of the ancient swamp. My mind swirled with hope and my thoughts were fueled by what my new life as a healthy person was going to be like. I felt elation in my decision, and just like that... I created a new future for myself and my family.

A New Language for a New Future

Nelsonian medicine ideology was about to turn my world right side up. Now that I had purchased a device of my own I began my studies. As I learned I released old ideas about what disease was and embraced new ways to solve mankind's oldest problem... illness.

As we take control of our health we expand our awareness from the limited knowledge of diseases within our organs, to understanding the organ's location and function within the body. Defining a few key words and phrases are important to getting us closer to the truth, and more importantly, closer to health.

When taking the quantum path on the journey to homeostasis, it's imperative to understand these three key players:

The Three Key Players

The Verbal Mind: The Verbal Mind is also known as the conscious mind. The Verbal Mind is doing all the talking, and for some of us it will chatter all night long preventing deep restorative sleep. It's your verbal mind that rationalizes, over thinks, and attempts to reduce information in order to get to symptom free living as quickly as possible. The verbal mind needs to be heard; however most of our verbal minds have under developed healing skills and over developed worrying skills. The verbal mind has limited experience with interfacing with the SUPERconscious mind and the Body Electric.

The SUPERconscious Mind: This part of the human mind remains a mystery to the scientific community and for years has been referred to as the unconscious or subconscious mind. This part of the human mind is not "un" conscious, as if it doesn't exist, and it's not "sub" conscious, as if it were less than. This part of you is so opposite to that concept that we call it the SUPERconscious.

The SUPERconscious Mind goes beyond the boundaries of your physical body and includes all of the subtle bodies that make up you the human being. For the sake of your wellness, understand that this part of yourself is the largest part of you. A subtle body is not seen with the naked eye, but it's always with you. Subtle bodies include the emotional subtle body, the mental subtle body, and the electromagnetic field surrounding the physical body. All of your life's experiences have been recorded by the SUPERconscious Mind. Good, bad, or indifferent this subtle information plays in the background of your existence. Your SUPERconscious Mind knows why there is pain. It knows why you're sick.

The powers of the mind have been well documented by the Princeton Engineering Anomalies Research (PEAR).[5] Consciousness has been proven through the Observer Effect. The term "Observer Effect" means that the act of observing, watching, or looking actually influences that which we observe. The observer effect is quantum physics proof that we create what we focus on.

Humans have always had a connection between mind and spirit. It's an undeniable force. Reductionist science's approach of the double blind placebo effect is to prevent every mind involved in the research from influencing the results, further supporting the proof of the powers of the mind.

Space or the ocean floor are considered the vast frontiers yet to be explored, by mainstream thought. Truth be known, the most vast frontier to be explored is *the human mind*.

The Body Electric: Brain waves and heartbeats are electrical. The nerves running throughout your body are conduits for electrical impulses which control your muscles. This is the power of the electrical moving you through existence. This is the Body Electric. Let us start at the beginning with the atom.

Richard Feynman, Nobel Laureate, Physics[6] gave us a simple explanation when he stated:

"I... a universe of atoms, an atom in the universe."

Desire Dubounet gives us a more in depth explanation in *Electroceuticals:*[7]

"In fifth grade we are all taught that our bodies are made of atoms. Atoms are made of electrons in the outer shell and since electrons never touch, they repel, atoms never touch. So nothing touches anything and drugs work thru energetic field interaction. In fact all of biology is field interaction. In nature the electrons are

moved into energetic orbits by photons where light thru the complex process of photosynthesis make the electrons move into higher energetic orbits that create high energy electrons in carbohydrates that are used to make energy ATP in the body."

My simpler understanding is that each and every person has within them a galaxy of 100,000,000,000 (100 billion) cells. Our verbal minds can not fathom the complexity of each of these cells.

Within each cell is an electron, a proton, the mitochondria and a large amount of empty space.[8] The mitochondria is a tiny power plant and is described as "the powerhouse of the cell" or "the energy currency of life." This is because it generates most of the cell's supply of adenosine triphosphate or ATP. ATP is a source of energy.[9]

The study of this energy or electrochemistry deals with the interaction between electrical energy and chemical change.[10] The Body Electric starts with electrochemistry and it's teaching us that biology is electrical in nature.[11] The domination of modern pharmaceutical funding in medical research in the United States, has left us unaware of the medical implications of electrical measurements. It's the investigation of this energetic field that better explains humans, as we are a complex open system.

To better explain a complex open system like the human body, we need to entertain a new idea: *the interaction of light with matter*. Light absorption is the key. Plants absorb light, or photons from the sun, called photosynthesis. The theory of interaction of light with matter is called the Quantum Electro Dynamics, or QED.

The proof of this theory came together in 1982 with **Promorpheus**; which was Professor Nelson's discovery of the Quantum Electro Dynamic field. His findings shed light on the truth of biology. The Quantum Electro Dynamic field, or QED tells us that *"any small (quantum) change in matter will release or absorb a photon."*[12] The Quantum Electro Dynamic field gives us the ability to describe the photon electron interaction. Like twinkling stars in a clear night's sky, I imagine our cells within each of us also twinkle with the releasing and absorbing of these photons.

The human body is a natural solar electrical power station, gaining energy via the interactions of photons. Professor Nelson explains in **Promorpheus** that electrons are either absorbing photons into the outer electrons (going into a higher quantic state) or releasing photons from the outer electrons (going into a lower quantic state). The relationship of the human body's 100,000,000,000 (one hundred billion) cells with all of those high energy outer electrons further supports our bio-electrical nature.

When we eat, our bodies use the converted carbohydrate high energy of photons from the food. These "high energy outer electrons" are used to make ATP and ADP. ADP is short for adenosine diphosphate, a group of molecules (called nucleotides) linked together with the function of transferring the energy from ATP and storing it for later use. ATP and ADP are the needed compounds of life, and are examples of covalent bonds.[13] Covalent bonds supply us the energy we need to stay alive. Living things use ATP like a battery, the ATP gives up energy when it loses its phosphorus group to form ADP, the food energy stored in the mitochondria convert the ADP back to ATP.[14]

The Body Electric gains these high energy covalent bonds with their outer electrons. The quality of our energy depend on the energy state of the covalent bonds. **Professor *Nelson shares the secrets to the proper energy states of the outer electrons: "the secret rests in the wisdom of nature*.**" The Quantum Electro Dynamic Field (QED) revels that the energy state of a plant grown in nature and a petrochemical substance from a pharmaceutical are different.[15] Plants use sunlight to convert ADP to ATP, petrochemicals don't.

When faced with a stopped heart a doctor uses electric stimulation to save the day! Why? Because you are a Body Electric! Every beat of your heart, each and every breath, the release of photons sends the pulse of life into the wonderful inner workings of the brain, igniting the Body Electric. The electrically charged brain waves deep within the brain signal the release of natural body substances like neurotransmitters and hormones into the blood stream. The endocrine system takes its cues from these electrical signals, sending them throughout the body to complete its many processes; like how shiny your hair is, how well your digestion works, or how well your toenails grow.

In Robert Becker's book, *The Body Electric* we're given an intriguing account of our bio-electrical selves. In 1985 this book introduced the idea that we are electrical in nature. Becker's exciting research and discoveries lead us to the doorway of a world where regenerating organs with electricity is possible.

Unfortunately, it's the Body Electric that has been left unattended and tossed aside in favor of using drugs for suppression of symptoms. Symptoms are cries for help. The Body Electric is completely ignored when it attempts requesting help via symptoms. Ignored until the heart stops and only then, in that life or death moment doctors are reminded to utilize the Body Electric. The Body Electric is so important that with God willing and a jolt of electricity that heart will restart and a life will be saved.

The SUPERconscious Mind interfaces with your Body Electric. When the SUPERconscious Mind and the Body Electric interface, the truth of what is making an individual go out of homeostasis begins to be revealed. This is bio resonance, and this is EXACTLY what Professor Nelson's devices resulted in being able to do. In my opinion this is why they're imperative for anyone hoping to take the journey back to wellness.

This is exactly what I experienced when I began the journey of real communication with my body. I listened and I used the information wisely, I took personal responsibility for lifestyle choices, I retrained my stress often and eventually the prize of homeostasis was attainable for me. This is exciting news! It's why those who know this technology and those who have been helped by it call it "Tomorrow's Medicine."

It's so important that I will say it again... on the road to wellness one must understand and respond to the messages of The Verbal Mind, The SUPERconscious Mind, and The Body Electric. Once their communication is established and all are heard, a new process of healing begins.

Tomorrow's Medicine and Today's Problem

Let's go deeper into what Professor Nelson's devices actually are and exactly how they can help Multiple Chemical Sensitivity (MCS), Chemical Intolerance (CI), Environmental Illness (EI) or Idiopathic Environmental Intolerance (IEI) individuals. Nelson's devices are registered as Biofeedback. Biofeedback is the designation the FDA[16] gives to a medical device that measures the body's physiological parameters. Amps, volts, and resistance are examples of physiological parameters. Once these electrical measurements are known, they can then be used to determine the electrical activity of all other organs within that body. This is called electrophysiology.[17]

Electrophysiology is:

- The study of the electrical properties of biological cells and tissues.

- Involved with measurements of voltage change or electric current on a wide variety of scales from a single protein to a whole organ like the brain.

- Electrophysiological readings have specific names:
  - Electrocardiography for the heart.
  - Electroencephalography for the brain.
  - Electrocorticography from the cerebral cortex.
  - Electromyography for the muscles.
  - Electrooculography for the eyes.
  - Electroretinography for the retina.
  - Electroantennography for the olfactory receptors in arthropods.

- Audiology for the auditory system.
- Electrocochleography for the cochlea.

Electrophysiology biofeedback interfaces with the Body Electric. With a traditional biofeedback device the client works with the conscious mind (The Verbal Mind) to manipulate and control an organ that is normally an automatic body function (such as blood pressure, heart rate, and muscle tension).

Biofeedback technology has advanced tremendously and today's new science of quantum physics gives way to a much more evolved device. A device that is referred to as *Quantum Biofeedback* in American vernacular and *Bio Resonance* in other countries, both are electrophysiological applications. Quantum Biofeedback is going one giant step further than traditional biofeedback as it accesses the SUPERconscious Mind and allows it to interface with the Body Electric.

The word quantum is defined as "any of the very small increments or parcels into which many forms of energy are subdivided."[18] In the case of biofeedback, *Quantum Biofeedback* measures the body's most subtle and smallest bits of information. This information is referred to as **resonance**. The SUPERconscious Mind and the Body Electric work together to resolve and eventually return all systems to **homeostasis** with the cooperation and participation of The Verbal Mind. These Quantum Biofeedback devices leave traditional biofeedback in the distant past with this quantum tool from tomorrow.

To delve even deeper, Nelson's Quantum Biofeedback devices enable the body to give and receive information. This information is in the form of stimulus, response, correct and re-stimulation, and it all works together to normalize and stabilize the Body Electric. This is done using the world's largest medical software. This software is one of many things that makes Professor Nelson's devices special and because it's placed on a cybernetic loop that allows it to perform at biological speeds.

Quoted from the software's opening video:

"This is the world's largest medical software, it is also the first on a cybernetic loop allowing the system to not only detect energetic aberrations but to correct them at biological speeds.
Speeds in excess of 1000th of a second."
-Professor William Nelson

In simple terms, the Quantum Biofeedback device works together with the software, (which is programmed with over 13,000 potential stressors), to ask the Body Electric via the SUPERconscious mind, "does this stressor give you stress?" and the body responds with, "yes, no, or maybe." This process is performed three times to assure accuracy. The cybernetic loop sends back a correcting frequency to retrain the body to better handle the stress which was detected. **These are very summarized and simplified explanations, but it's necessary to clarify the differences between traditional biofeedback and Quantum Biofeedback.**

The FDA makes no distinction between the psycho-physiology biofeedback devices of forty years ago and today's far more encompassing device using electrophysiological Quantum Biofeedback technology. This is like having the 1930's phone systems that required an operator to dial a number for you and your smart phone being placed into the same designation as "communication devices." Today in the United States all medical devices are under FDA regulations. The FDA regulates a broad range of medical devices from artificial hearts to tongue depressors, biofeedback falls somewhere in the middle.[19] The FDA classifies Professor Nelson's biofeedback devices as Class 2 medical devices.

The first electrophysiology biofeedback system device, was developed by Professor Nelson and registered with the FDA October 13, 1989 following twenty years of research in the field of energetic medicine and bio-resonance. But what does bio-resonance mean? To be resonant is to be in a sympathetic vibration and repeatedly reflected awareness. Professor Nelson gives a simple example of two kids playing catch together, the tossing of the ball back and forth to each other is an example of repeated reflected awareness. In electrophysiological biofeedback, bioresonance refers to the body's cells and their perfect state of being. Resonance is a song sung perfectly in tune.

Today with advances in hardware and software, Professor Nelson has continued to enhance and develop the electrophysiological biofeedback systems. The QXCI, EPFX, SCIO, INDIGO, The Educator and the EDUCTOR. For those who want to know more Professor Nelson has published A Professional Clinical Evaluation of the QQC Electronic Tongue (http://youtu.be/mHamMVOhi2A). This video contains scientific history and a more in depth explanation as well as a review of the process that validates energetic medicine. Now that you've been introduced to the good guys of wellness, it's time to met their opponents.

Stress: The Askew Serial Killer

If you're getting ill for any reason, it's always important that you understand your true enemy. Enemy number one is STRESS. Stress the prime serial killer our society allows to run rampant through our lives killing millions of people each year, and yet we make jokes about it. Our society's perception of stress is off center, and severely askew to the danger of this uncontrolled killer. Everyone needs to understand that stress **is dangerous**. For chemical sensitive people, a knowledge of how to retrain the body to better handle the effects of stress is the skill you need to master for the prize of homeostasis.

In the early decades of the twentieth century, Hans Selye, a Hungarian doctor spent decades observing patients. These patients appeared to be in good health but with the exception of a few symptoms. Once these symptoms were addressed, and the patient was symptom free, the patient would later develop a disease. Dr. Selye noted this period of "pre disease" as *stress*.

Dr. Selye's medical practice and legendary work on stress gives us a simple explanation on how to stop disease at its earliest stages and even prevent it from forming. Dr. Selye used his powers of observation and with an uncensored scientific mind he gave humanity a glowing achievement of truth in medicine: **Pain is the emergency alarm system of your body, not the enemy.** Like a car alarm, pain's purpose is to get your attention. Instead of figuring out why the alarm has gone off, we ignore the alarm and suppress it with medicine made of petrochemicals.

"Stress in health and disease is medically, sociologically, and philosophically the most meaningful subject for humanity that I can think of."

- Dr. Hans Selye

To understand this different way of being truly healthy you have to start with Hans Selye's flow chart on the "Pathway of Disease." This flow chart below may seem awkward to you at first, but it's actually very simple. Simple is good. Once you get this, the rest is easy!

Hans Selye's Pathway of Disease

Start at Health →
Then enters the stressor (toxin, pathogen, injury, etc) →
First stage reached: the alarm stage.

ALARM STAGE

- Symptoms at first are related to the stressor, later the dysfunction.
- Examples of symptoms: pain, swelling, bloating, redness, lack of vitality, mental fog, depression, and more...
- Examples of dysfunction: constipation, high blood pressure, hormonal imbalances, and more
- Symptoms are the alarm, not the enemy.

If stress is ignored, suppressed, or continues for any reason →
Second stage reached: the adaptation stage. →

ADAPTATION STAGE

- Symptoms leave as the body *adapts* to the stress.
- Distress and disease go deeper.
- You can have no symptoms, yet still be very sick.

BEING SYMPTOM FREE IS NOT AN INDICATOR OF HEALTH!

If stress is still ignored, suppressed, or continues for any reason →

Then you enter the third stage

EXHAUSTION STAGE

- In the exhaustion phase the stressors begin to burden the weakest organs.
- Within the exhaustion phase there are three levels...

1) FUNCTIONAL
- First the stressors affect the weakest organ's function.
- If stressors continue you move into the organic level.

2) ORGANIC
- Organic means a disease originates from the organ due to the disturbance of function.
- The weak organ starts to swell or shrink.
- If stressors continue you move into the final level...

3) DEATH
- Cellular death
- Organ death
- Organ system failure
- Body death

When stress disrupts the natural state of your cells, it creates confusion and sets the stage for disease to occur. When your cells are brought back to their natural state, any illness that was in progress or about to make progress is impeded, stopped, and possibly given a U-turn. When you look at illness in this way, you will take the first step toward wellness. When your cells are kept in their natural state they're better able to stay out of the confused state of disease and illness. It's imperative to shift the way you think about your body and your health. It takes a paradigm shift.

That new paradigm is simple:

Homeostasis = Wellness
Stress = Illness

Dr. Selye's flow chart spells it out, being symptom free is not an indicator of health. Professor Nelson designed a new type of medicine around Hans Selye's life's work. The Nelson Method of Medicine is steeped with Dr. Selye's wisdom and infused with the genius of Professor Nelson's **Promorpheus** and the Quantum Electro Dynamics, or QED (reminder that the QED is Professor Nelson's theory of the interaction of light with matter). This gives us a new way back to wellness and true health; a return to homeostasis. This is why Quantum Biofeedback becomes an amazing tool for health and wellness!

"Neither the prestige of your subjects and the power of your instruments nor the extent of your planning can substitute for the originality of your approach and the keenness of your observation.

-Dr. Hans Selye
(The motto at the entrance to his institute.)

132

How does A New Science Help?

Side note: The following italicized titles are from the manufacturer's website www.qxsubspace.com, for Professor Nelson's devices. Reprinted with permission, these titles express the biofeedback devices capabilities precisely. The rest is my humble observations of safety and efficiency from my many years of experience. (See Resources for more on safety and efficacy)

#1) ***Detection of Stress and Reduction of Stress:*** This is simple and needed for everyone, especially people with MCS, CI, EI, and IEI! Chemicals create stresses which are both detectable and measurable. This type of stress confuses the natural state of your cells and makes the CI, EI, and MCS person a mess. The EI and IEI sufferer experiences stress from the environment which is also detectable and measurable. I was able to retrain my body to better handle the many variations of environmental stress.

Regular retraining releases the cells from their toxic burden. For me this means less down time being sick in bed or in pain. With regular retraining over time, I was able to, on my own, better manage my body's reactions to toxins. With patience and persistence in using the device I stopped being so overwhelmed and devastated by every toxin around me. Regular retraining releases the cells from their toxic burden. I experienced this first hand.

#2) ***Muscular Re-Education from Injury, Muscle Weakness, or Dystonia:*** For the multiple chemical sensitive person chemicals make the muscles weak (and maybe everyone's). Retraining helped me get my strength back.

Dystonia is caused by a neurological disorder stemming from the brain's basal ganglia which is when the muscles contract and hold the body in unnatural positions. This has happened to me with my toes since my late teens. My right foot was the worst, with the toes pulling up and pointing to the sky.

Since I started Quantum Biofeedback retraining my toes have been calm and no painful contractions have happened in the last ten years. I would like to note that during my first few years of working on my chemical stress a great deal of time was spent on retraining the basal ganglia. The basal ganglia was chosen by my *SUPERconsciousness* during my biofeedback sessions for many months.

#3) ***Healing of Trauma and Wounds:*** Using the Quantum Biofeedback device I've experienced my own healings of trauma. I've also observed my family, and my clients heal from trauma. On myself I observed a decades old injury with a raised scar soften and slowly flatten and fade into a line which is barely visible. I have also observed wounds heal considerably faster, and I'm often surprised at how quickly bruising fades when I use the Quantum Biofeedback device for that specific purpose.

#4) ***Pain Reduction Through M.E.N.S.:*** Quantum Bio-feedback offers simple pain reduction through Microcurrent [Transcutaneous] Electro Nerval Stimulation. M.E.N.S. is used for pain and to speed the healing of wounds; my own personal experience has shown it to be an exceptional performer as a pain reliever on a tendon and ligament injury. The gentle and extremely small electric current is sent into the body to the nerves. It's non invasive and drug free, with no harmful side effects, no petrochemical drugs, no needles... just pain reduction and faster recovery.

#5) ***Rectification of Charged Stability Imbalance and Redox Potential:*** We're going to begin working with some new concepts that include new terminology. The following are a few definitions taken from the "language" of Quantum Biofeedback.

Rectification - A score is assigned when specific information about an individual is fed into the biofeedback device and that information is analyzed within the program. This score is used to show the overall balance of your natural state. The lower the score the more correction is needed to return to homeostasis.

Charged stability imbalance - How to bring balance to the imbalanced and reduces the stress reaction to any physical, mental, or emotional stress that disturbs the body's homeostasis. This is the end result of a session, or the side effects if you want to give it more of a label. It happens when running the retraining programs chosen by the SUPERconscious for stability and balance of the Body Electric.

Redox - An abbreviation for "*red*uction *ox*idation". The quantum technology capabilities increase the body's potential to release oxidation from within the cell. Oxidation is the body's enemy. Oxidation to your cells is like rust to steel, it speeds up the aging process, and when combined with free radicals, over time, it results in organ damage. Oxidation left in the cell results in degenerative events like cancer and age related damage.

Environmental Illness sufferers have several program options with this technology. The environment offers many stress causing measurable frequencies that create aberrant waves within the human body. Several potential stressors can disrupt the natural electric flow of your cells including naturally occurring Earth phenomenon and man-made stressors. Other examples of disruptive environmental phenomenon are geopathic stress, electromagnetic stress from electric sources, including appliances, as well as energy from the sun, dying stars, cell phones, and human thoughts... and that's the short list.

Those with EI have been known to suffer to the point of living in the wilderness as far from civilization's electrical pulses as possible. I have observed the device detect and retrain a client's Body Electric to better handle the effects of stress from EMFs in the environment. In the next section EI/IEI sufferers will want to pay special attention to "Perverse Energy", which is a Chinese medical category for environmental factors that create stress within the Body Electric.

A New Method of Medicine

We've begun to define Quantum Biofeedback but how can it help the suffering? We have to understand a few simple new ideas of what health looks like. The statements below may seem complicated. Simply read over them, relax, read the next section, and come back to this section later if needed.

The following quotes on Nelsonian Medicine are reprinted with permission from Professor Nelson:

"Fractal and Chaos theory have taught us the complexity of humans. We must respect the whole individual not the reduction of their parts. A small flaw on any part might amplify a disease elsewhere."

"Health is ease of flow."

"A stressor blocks flow, stress is more than JUST personal stress."

"When the stressor or stressors weaken the defenses of the body, the weakest link of the body (from nature to nurture) is most prone to distress and thus disease."

*"Stress Reduction is **KEY** to medicine."*

The following five steps are the foundation of Nelsonian Medicine, based on Hans Selye's life work.

NELSONIAN MEDICINE[20]

FLOW OF TREATMENT AND CURE

1. Reduce or remove the cause of disease *(the stressor)*:

Major stress categories include:

- ❖ LACK OF AWARENESS OR KNOWLEDGE
- ❖ STRESS
- ❖ HEREDITY
- ❖ MENTAL FACTORS
- ❖ ALLERGY
- ❖ TOXICITY
- ❖ TRAUMA INJURY
- ❖ PATHOGENS
- ❖ PERVERSE ENERGY
- ❖ DEFICIENCY OR EXCESS OF NUTRITIENTS

2. Treat the organs effected or diseased.

3. Unblock the blockages to flow of life.

4. Reduce symptoms and all suffering naturally.

5. Treat constitutional and metabolic tendencies to disease patterns or habits.

Nelsonian medicine is very simple and safe. It empowers us to get well by reducing stress and retraining damaged organs. The combination of Nelsonian and Selye systems creates a safe, inexpensive, and effective new modern medicine. Western medicine is very complicated with undesirable and sometimes dangerous side effects, especially for the Chemical Intolerant individual.

Chapter Eleven

Living Proof

"Truth is what stands the test of experience."
~Albert Einstein~

I'm living proof Professor Nelson is correct. As I look back it's obvious that sharing what I've learned with you is my life's purpose. Showing others proof that there's another option, an option that works is my service to my fellow humans and to God. This is what I'm here to do. Forced up against the wall, I was blessed to be given no other choice to survive except to embrace this path.

Using the technology developed by Professor Nelson and choosing to follow a new paradigm of caring for myself, I overcame a chemical load, allergies, chronic inflammation, liver failure, and I released what I thought I knew from my education, medical information, society, and mainstream media. Instead I followed the innate wisdom of my body. Retraining my body's inflammation response to all hyper reactants worked and I was rewarded with improving health. For ten years I was my own researcher and through experience, observation, documentation, and surviving, I can offer verification to the soundness of Nelsonian Medicine by ultimately staying alive. I am proof we can take back our health and become well and vibrant once again without pharmaceutical drugs. It takes fearless commitment, critical thinking, and strong intuition... all normal human behaviors.

My gift to you is the **truth**. Nelsonian Medicine works **if** you take responsibility for your choices, use your critical thinking, and stop ignoring pain by numbing it with petrochemical based prescription drugs, alcohol, and street drugs. Instead listen to your pain as your body's cry for help.

Are your choices helping you overcome Multiple Chemical Sensitives (MCS) or are you heading towards Chemical Intolerance (CI)? I can assure you that continuing to do the same thing will get you the same results. Eventually the steroids turned on me and I found myself on Hans Selye's pathway to disease. Are you, or someone you know, on this pathway? Chances are your answer is yes. If so, change is **now**. Open your heart and mind, releasing all attachments to all outcomes. Suspend all beliefs in what *is*, and get ready for what can **be**...

Verification Through My Results

In this section I weave my personal story with the truth and simplicity of Nelsonian Medicine to help draw a more complete picture of what returning to homeostasis looks like. I'm going to show you exactly how I used Nelsonian Medicine's Flow of Treatment to bring myself from the brink of death back to being alive, healthy, and vibrant.

Following the Nelsonian Medicine Flow of Treatment and Cure I will illustrate its effectiveness by connecting my personal journey and training in Quantum Biofeedback to each Treatment and Cure category. Remember Professor Nelson's quote, *"When the stressor or stressors weaken the defenses of the body, the weakest link of the body (from nature to nurture) is most prone to distress and thus disease."* In each category we will point out the stressor in order to help everyone begin to identify their personal stressors.

#1) Reduce or Remove the Cause of Disease (the Stressor): The only way for me to reduce or remove the cause of disease was to remove myself from the entertainment industry. For decades I had been attempting to avoid chemicals in food and beauty products, but I couldn't escape them in the workplace. It was a sad day for me to request a retired card from I.A.T.S.E. Local 477, my trade union of fellow film makers. That was the day I had to face the truth of step one in Nelsonian Medicine: **"Remove the cause of disease."**

Major Stress Categories:

LACK OF AWARENESS or LACK OF KNOWLEDGE:
Five months after purchasing the SCIO/EDUCTOR I went to a Congress of Quantum Masters, held in Cabos San Lucas, Mexico. It was April of 2006. This was the three day training seminar with Professor Nelson that was included when I purchased my device. In order to travel I had to arrest the massive inflammatory response of my body. I was able to accomplish this using the device with my limited technical knowledge.

Shortly after arriving I saw four previous classmates from my beginner's class who didn't recognize me and walked right past me. When I stopped them to remind them of who I was, they were shocked! It had only been five months since they'd last seen me and they couldn't believe I had improved to the point of being unrecognizable. One of my classmates, Roxanne, a retired hospice nurse seemed to be the most surprised. They all confessed their surprise was due to the general belief of the group, that I was not going to make it five months earlier.

"We thought you were a goner!" they all exclaimed as they stood around me touching my hair and face and giving me hugs.

It felt great to surprise them with health. I had no idea how bad I had appeared to others. Roxanne later told me that back in December I had the gray death pallor in my face.

"I've helped people die for over twenty years Kristy, you were dying." she said to me. "I was concerned that you were going to have heart failure and so I was always nearby ready to do CPR for you."

Although her observations both comforted and alarmed me, I was touched by her sincerity and caring. In that moment I realized how sick I had been. It also confirmed my lack of awareness and that staying unaware was at my own peril. **Lack of Awareness is a stressor.**

STRESS: The June 6, 1983 Time Magazine cover declared stress as the country's leading health problem.[1] In 1994, research showed that 60% to 90% of doctors visits were stress related. Now in the year 2016, we continue to be a nation under stress.

My personal stress was as significant as the physical stress of my last big chemical exposure. During the next few years my daughter and her family made an exodus to an area hours away. My illness made working difficult, so unfortunately my home of twenty years was forfeited to the bank. I had to sacrifice almost all my worldly possessions; forced to give away pets, knick knacks, and furniture. Additionally, my acute sensitivity to chemicals increased the amount of stress to my body.

I continued my weekly sessions with the SCIO/EDUCTOR for chemicals and I was also addressing all my SUPERconscious choices for stress in general. I know these retrainings were instrumental in surviving these hard times without being sicker, and hysterically crying all the time. I also kept my immediate family on regular SUPERconscious stress retraining sessions as well. Although we were all under personal stress through those grueling years, we managed to stay well and in homeostasis, despite the odds.

Stress is personal and relative to the individual. Stress is aberrant energy misplaced in a body. It doesn't matter whether that stress is within the physical body due to a flu virus, or in the emotional body from the pain of a loss, or in the mental body due to over working or being mentally exhausted. There could even be family stress from over worry or social stress from an event. These are all just a few examples of personal stress that comes from things other than chemicals or the environment.

If your body is responding to chemicals in a negative way rejoice! Your body is alarming you to stress and with Professor Nelson's devices retraining your body's ability to handle that stress is now possible! Remember, Professor Nelson's Quantum Biofeedback devices empower us to get well **by retraining the body to better handle stress.**

Effective stress management is one of the keys to achieving and maintaining good health. Effective stress management is more than taking a day off or taking up a hobby, it requires a new science and a new way of thinking about wellness.

HEREDITY: As I mentioned earlier, stress accounts for 95% of diseases. You may have been wondering what happened to the other 5%. That 5% is given over to genetics. Which is why understanding DNA is important. DNA is called the "molecule of life" for a reason. It's the blueprint of our physical structure. It contains all the information about how you, as a living thing, will look and function.

Dr. Fritz-Albert Popp is the founder of the International Institute of Biophysics in Neuss (1996), Germany, an international network of 19 research groups from 13 countries involved in biophoton research and coherence systems in biology and our DNA.

Dr Fritz Popp says, *"DNA is our genetic code of life; it is how we reproduce and replicate cells. Our DNA can be distorted and trigger disease. Light in the DNA is coherent in health. DNA is the information center of the cell, and this light consequently appears to emerge from the DNA and pass on the communication of the DNA to the cell association and therefore to control the cell association through the information in the light. The vital thread of DNA can be damaged in many different ways, UV radiation, ionizing radiation, EMF and electrical radiation and by a vast* **number of toxic and chemical substances and processes. Their destructive effects can cause part of the DNA to be torn out or incorrectly inserted and its strands can be broken apart and destroyed.**[2]

Our body employs the appropriate repair depending on the damage, and we can carry on living, ideally. When our body is constantly exposed to these destructive effects it has to work harder and sometimes it just cannot cope with the ever-increasing amounts of destructive energy thrown at it."[3]

Professor Nelson states in **Promorpheus**; *"DNA is a receiver and transmitter of laser light."* **Damaged DNA and genetic defects are stressors.**

I have personally experienced retraining the DNA replication, and observed the course of expression of an improper genetic tendency <u>change direction</u>, when I was working to overcome the chemical exposure using the SCIO/EDUCTOR. I will be expanding on this experience in another book, as more time progresses with my good health intact. I want to observe this a little longer. I only share it now so you can understand how surprised I was with this delightful side effect of running retraining programs for DNA whenever my SUPERconscious requested it. **Improperly inherited genetic tendencies are a stressor.**

MENTAL FACTORS: Mental factors are another form of stress that affects one's health. After my SCIO/EDUCTOR training in Cabos San Lucas I worked on myself and practiced on everybody who showed any interest. People came through the door in a constant stream and I became faster at running the device. As I learned and became more proficient that first year I successfully helped others.

Unfortunately, as I mentioned earlier, I ran out of money. I had no idea that in order to follow this path and become well, I would eventually go through all my savings, my retirement, the equity in my house and eventually the house itself during the great bank bailout of 2008. However, in 2006 I had an intention for success as I concentrated on regaining my health and becoming certified as a Quantum Biofeedback Specialist. By the end of 2006 by shear determination I was officially certified, trained, and qualified to charge clients. It was time to start earning an income. To my heartbreak all those people I freely gave sessions to, all those people I helped didn't return with cash. They didn't refer their friends or family. They all disappeared and I felt abandoned. This turn of events really confused me.

When I ran myself on the device it showed that I was in resonance with the frequency of 'apathy.' Apathy is a Chemical

Intolerance (CI) symptom and the bullet in the gun of Multiple Chemical Sensitivity (MCS). Apathy is how the sick MCS and CI sufferers get shoved to the side. Ultimately, I came to understand what my SUPERconscious was telling me through the Quantum Biofeedback: I <u>allowed</u> apathy by not setting clear boundaries with people. In retrospect, I see that apathy and depression were overriding common sense behavior choices.

Detoxification and retraining of these less than desirable mental factors was accelerated using the programs with Professor Nelson's Quantum Biofeedback device. Until I started to feel better I didn't realize how ill I was. It took getting past apathy and working through other less than desirable mental factors such as anger and confusion, that were not supporting my healing. With regular stress reduction, using Essential Oils and the practice of saying and writing affirmations given to me by the program, my mental clarity and joy returned!

Writing, saying and thinking positive affirming sentences is a simple way to retrain my mental body and correct limiting, self defeating thoughts. But like the gym you have to do the work to get results. For years I have used positive affirmations to develop a mental tone of positivism. The software offers several affirmations each session to enhance this type of mental retraining. **Mental factors blocking the flow of energy are stressors** and I have experienced relief from negative repeating thoughts with regular Quantum Biofeedback retraining and commitment to making better life style choices.

ALLERGY: All allergies, known or unknown, create inflammation within the body. What an allergy doctor calls an allergy I will refer to as a *hyper reaction* since I'm not a doctor. Inflammation takes us out of homeostasis and is our body crying out for help, asking us to remove it from the stress. Yes! Allergies are stressors. Even with a confirmed medical diagnosis for my allergy with toluene aka methyl benzene it did not change my suffering.

When I began to use the SCIO/EDUCTOR it was no

surprise when toluene and benzene, chlorine, mold and dust would show up throughout my sessions for retraining in the hyper reactant (allergy) and detox programs. In the past these allergies would interrupt my daily life and all I could do was remove myself from the offender. Now after ten years of the SCIO/EDUCTOR and eighteen years with Essential Oils I can be among the offenders. Although briefly for some and a little longer for others, as long as I'm using my solutions I'm not thrown on the floor or running out the door. I'm now able to tolerate my stressors rather than fall ill. This has allowed me to go out and be with people once again.

The SCIO/EDUCTOR also was revealing other sources of the inflammation plaguing my body. The SCIO/EDUCTOR's software listed this inflammatory response to be also from many of the foods that were on my personal hyper reactants list. It surprised me to see that many foods I was eating were on my personal hyper reactants list. Foods that are the base of our modern diet. Simple foods like soy, rice, wheat, corn, canola and cottonseed oil.

I continued to retrain the toluene allergy and the hyper reaction to grains and oils. Over the years I have been able to safely add back into my diet (on a limited basis) oats, barley, and kamut, an ancient wheat. I continue to experience a hyper reaction symptom of acid reflux and inflammation when I eat canola oil, cottonseed oil, corn, and rice.

In my opinion, a chemical sensitive person does not need an allergy test to confirm the reaction to a chemical as an allergy. A chemical sensitive person needs help detoxing. Regular hyper reactant retraining with the device has helped me to become less inflamed and reactionary to my known and unknown allergies, allowing me an increase in the quality of my life. **Allergies controlled with drugs or not, known and not known are a stressor.**

TOXICITY: Toxicity shows up in many different guises. Toxicity, or a buildup of chemical poisons called "toxic load," can affect the neurological, immune, and endocrine systems, as well as skin, bones, intestines and liver. In my opinion toxicity can affect us beyond only the physical body and intrude upon the subtle bodies as well.

Petroleum based chemicals are man-made and are toxic to everyone's cells. I cannot tolerate petroleum based chemicals and my reactions are immediate. Everyone's reactions may not be immediate though; some reactions may take twenty years to present themselves. Do we really have to get cancer before we wake up to the dangers of benzene toxicity?

At a molecular level our cells know the truth. Anti-inflammatory medications are not made from plants, they're made from a carbon of the mother solvent, benzene. A pharmaceutical steroid is not made of a flower molecule; a steroid is made of a benzene molecule. The benzene molecule harmed my cellular receptor sites. Eventually steroid medication turned on me and became part of the toxic mix within my sick body, creating a life threatening toxic load.

An emergency room doctor explained to me that everyone is born with a *"chemical savings account"* known as the blood brain barrier (BBB). The BBB is a tightly woven physical barrier that protects the brain from the blood stream. Therefore, nothing that gets into the bloodstream, like an infection or a virus, can get past the barrier into the brain. Every time we ingest chemicals in the food or the air, we are deducting from this chemical savings account of the blood brain barrier, an account we can only withdraw from. We can never make a deposit into this account and once the balance is zero the blood brain barrier is bankrupt and we will die.

He went on to explain that my body took a major withdrawal from its blood brain barrier chemical savings account when I had my chemical emergencies and I was now at risk; one more withdrawal like that and I would be "over drawn and bankrupt."

This was such a scary scenario for me that I had to know

more about my chemical enemy. I learned that benzene dissolves sulfur and iodine, minerals necessary for life. Why use benzene based food additives in our food when it dissolves sulfur and iodine? What purpose is there for the body to have sulfur dissolved when it's considered a building block of life? Years later, as I began to work with the Quantum Biofeedback devices, I would understand more fully the connection between endocrine imbalances and stress from food additives, beauty products, household products, and pharmaceuticals based in benzene science.

Within the device is a homotoxicology program designed to stimulate detoxification. This program provides a magnetic electrical pulse that will shake up the benzene molecules and other free radicals along with heavy metals and increase their excretion from the body.

Running this program regularly made a big difference in my quality of life and kept me from making a final and terminal withdrawal from my BBB bank. With the help of the homotoxicology program I began my ascent back into homeostasis and stopped the sliding descent into death. **All toxins are a stressor.**

TRAUMA / INJURY: Any instance of being injured, harmed or damaged creates stress. Physical injury or any deeply disturbing experience or event in life can be stressful and lingering.

Chemicals made from the mother solvent in all their form, are traumatic to your cells and injuring your organs, making them swell. Retraining this molecular trauma was of paramount importance for my recovery from Chemical Intolerance.

The first training class I experienced with the SCIO/EDUCTOR and learning Quantum Biofeedback was incredibly accurate although at first confusing. The device opened a program called "Trauma Repair" and giving me a SUPERconscious choice telling me to retrain "Frost bite injury" this was odd since I reside in the tropics. Also during this session several industrial chemicals were also showing up in the detox panel to be retrained out of my body. Later when I researched these chemicals I would learn that when exposed to one of them without protective respiratory gear will damage the lungs as if they have suffered frostbite. After this first training experience I began to breathe deeper and my awe for this technology increased ten fold.

Since starting this book I have had two physical injuries. The first injury was to both legs from a fall onto asphalt, leaving me scrapped and both knees badly bruised. The second injury a few years later was a high ankle sprain. Both injuries resulted in laying me flat on my back and not able to move or care for myself for several days.

Applying the solutions in my book got me through those two painful and frightening experiences without the need to seek out emergency room treatment and chemical medication. With Chemical Intolerance (CI) I've learned emergency rooms are a dangerous place for me and there isn't much they can offer since I can't take the steroids nor most of the benzene based medications. Before all these solutions entered my life, our last visits to an emergency room was for my son's broken arm and later a broken nose. Both visits resulted in me being ill for several weeks from the many disinfectants and floor cleaning chemicals used in emergency rooms.

That first injury took about a month to return to normal. My legs and knees were bruised and painful and kept me from kneeling down directly on them for many months. However I was walking without pain and could bend my knees with no problem. No broken bones. I got through the experience with no pain medications. I rested and used ice, and all my solutions mentioned thus far.

The same goes for the second injury, a much more extensive injury and once again I was supported with these solutions. This time I had a new friend who was at the end stages of the same type of ankle injury. When I sent her pictures of my three week old injury she expressed surprise at my progress. Her five year old injury was still resulting in re-injury and a continued need to wrap, ice and nurse the same ankle.

The technology of the SCIO/EDUCTOR has given me remarkable results for injuries whether from a fall, a toxin or from the emotions trauma can leave on us as we recover. **Injury and trauma can be stressors that may linger for years.**

**PATHOGENS**: One of the biggest problems I have with chemicals is the lowered immune response to pathogens. I have learned first hand the immune system's response to bacteria, fungus, virus, spirochetes, prions, protozoa, worms, and amoebas is greatly reduced when the organs are full of petroleum chemicals.

Before my Quantum Biofeedback journey I received a life changing diagnosis of first stage cervical cancer in 1992. Heather gave me a copy of Hulda Clark's *Cure for all Cancers*. Hulda Clark found that the life cycle of the sheep liver fluke easily flourished in the human liver saturated with isopropyl alcohol, another offspring of the mother solvent. She opened my mind to the presence of pathogens in our bodies that went beyond virus, bacteria, and candida. She blew my mind with her case studies of people being cleared of horrible diseases after they cleaned up the toxins and rid themselves of parasites and toxic molds. Using Hulda's parasite cleanse as my guideline, I started my first parasite cleanse and was quite shocked by the large spaghetti like tapeworm I purged. There was no doubt, parasites were an issue for me, keeping my immune system over worked and allowing a cancer virus to gain strength.

In my beginner's SCIO/EDUCTOR training I was a test subject for the class. My instructor did some zapping[4] for parasites. The SCIO/EDUCTOR was showing I was in resonance with several different varieties. Before my session was over I felt that odd sensation in my mid section and a surprising need to have a bowel movement. My reward from his SCIO/EDUCTOR session was several different worm bodies left behind in the toilet.

Worms play a bigger part in our lives than we realize.

Contrary to common belief, worms do exist in America and you don't need to travel to a third world country to get infected. When a body carries a worm load, the liver and kidneys must process your wastes <u>and</u> the worm's waste. Entertaining worms is not in your body's best interest, and it's a must to keep them evicted and unwelcome every day. With this knowledge it becomes necessary to have supreme toilet hygiene (not only yours but anyone who may handle your food), as well as a regular fall and spring practice of parasite cleansing, daily ingestion of Essential Oils, and run worm zapping programs through the SCIO/EDUCTOR.

I have learned that the best course of action for a pathogen is a strong immune system. With a virus or unfriendly bacteria I take decisive action and strike immediately by running appropriate programs within the SCIO/EDUCTOR and consuming the recommended Essential Oils, along with other solutions. I have found this to be an effective defense when I must deal with pathogens.

All pathogens visible or microscopic are stressors running rampantly though so many of us, creating an unknown cesspool of stress within.

PERVERSE ENERGY*:* Environmental Illness folks are vindicated with this category. Perverse Energy is a Chinese Medicine term referring to the affect of the environment and its effects on the body. This includes wind, dampness, heat, and cold; as well as other environmental concerns like geopathic stress, electromagnetic frequencies (EMF) stress from power stations, electric power tools, cell phones, and electrical appliances. When weather causes people to become too hot or too cold they're experiencing the effects of Perverse Energy. These subtle energies within the environment can be measured and they are stressors.

During my self-run SCIO/EDUCTOR sessions the term "geopathic stress" came up several times. Geopathic stress is defined as *"The energy emitted by the earth at a specific location on the surface, which affects the human body function."* Historically this energy was detected through the use of dowsing, which is an ancient and simple process for divining ground water.

Ground water has been tied to the existence of geopathic stress. An article in *The Current Science* from March 10, 2010 *"Geopathic stress: a study to understand its nature using Light Interference Technique"* studies light based measuring methods in order to provide scientific support to the realities of geopathic stress. This geopathic stress energy can be beneficial, but some of it's highly destructive and can create disturbing energies within your Body Electric which can lead to degenerative diseases like cancer.

In order to find out exactly where the "walls" of detrimental geopathic stress existed, I had my home measured by a dowser highly experienced with measuring geopathic stress. The easiest cure for geopathic stress is simply moving yourself out of these areas. When I moved my furniture out of these areas my energy increased and degeneration pain diminished. Using regular Quantum Biofeedback retraining helped turn down the "buzzy energy" I could feel in my body from some of the geopathic stress walls.

There are some cures that can be added to the environment to help tame some geopathic stress energy. One that I used successfully was the placement of one foot wide copper staples into the ground outside my home. I placed one of these copper staples outside the house into the ground where the dowser had detected a geopathic "wall" into and out of the house. As soon as I placed them into the ground there was noticeable energy shift for me. The dowser came back and remeasured those areas and told me the copper staples had taken two foot wide walls and reduced them to about six inches wide. Feng Shui is another methodology that can be applied to reducing the affects of geopathic stress in a space. I also use another methodology discussed in Chapter 12.

Electromagnetic frequencies (EMF) are another source of irritation and energy that can be disruptive to the human body. The EPA has classified Magnetic fields as a Class 3 carcinogen.

Magnetic Field sources:

- Emanate from main power meter of home
- Electric clock radios

EMF sources :

- Electric fields emanate from anything electrical.
- Power Lines
- Metal Plumbing in some Older Structures
- Wireless Communications Mast Base Stations
- Wireless Networks or WiFi
- Cell Phones
- Cordless Phones
- Smart Meters
- Electric wiring in the home.
- Microwave Ovens
- Computers

EMF sources can come from high frequency electrical pulses coming out about six feet from an electrical pole. They also emanate from the wall near electrical outlets. These pulses come out about six inches and go around the room where the wire runs through the wall. Metal box springs up against this field can conduct this electric pulse and can disrupt sleep. I have placed my bed in the center of the room many feet away from the electric outlets and removed clocks, radios, TVs and cell phones away from my sleeping area. This was enough for me to sleep better, however other EI sufferers may need to be more proactive.

Proactive means examining every source of potential entry of these fields and remove the sleeping area as far from the field as possible. Look for electrical sources on the other side of the wall where you sleep or other areas you spend time.

Mother Earth offers help with two crystals Tourmaline and Rose Quartz. These two crystals help with dispersing some electromagnetic energy in the environment. I place these crystals around my computer.

"EMFs can reduce the ability of white blood cells to kill tumor cells, affect our reproduction, create problems with cell growth and affect the CNS (Central Nervous System) and the brain, which can lead to cancer and cancer related problems" says Professor Ross Adey, one of the most respected bio-electromagnetic researchers in the world."[5]

The IARC (International Agency for Research on Cancer) cites evidence for a link between humans and EMFs as possible carcinogenic[6] to humans based on epidemiological studies of childhood leukemia as well as a small increase in brain tumors of electrical workers.

The findings of EMF studies on laboratory animals is that they:

- Affect cell growth regulation...consistent with tumor formation.
- Increase tumor incidence.
- Alter gene transcriptional processes, the natural defense response of T-Lymphocytes and other cellular processes, related to the development and control of cancers.
- Affect neuroendocrine and psychosexual responses.[7]

There are other perverse low frequencies called extremely low frequency (ELF) and extreme extreme low frequencies (EELF) some also call this very low frequencies (VLF). High frequencies or low frequencies these are all out of sync with our Body Electric's natural harmonic pulse.

In 2008 The Bio-initiative Report[8] was released with alarming evidence. This report was based on international research and a public policy initiative to give an overview of what is known about the biological effects that occur at low intensity electromagnetic fields.

Some of the fields reviewed were:

- ELF (extremely low frequency)
- EMF (electromagnetic fields)
- Radio frequency
- Microwave radiation

The report on these various electro magnetic fields and their effects on human health associated with exposure from emissions were:

- Childhood Leukemia
- Brain Tumors
- Genotoxic Effects
- Neurological Effects, Neuro-degenerative Disease
- Immune System Deregulation
- Allergic and Inflammatory Responses
- Breast Cancer
- Miscarriage
- Cardiovascular Effects

Two decades of research supporting the same health concerns coming from these man-made frequencies, frequencies that should not be taken lightly. Those sensitive to pick up on these troubling stressful energies need compassion and a safe place to live. We need more radio free zones like the one in Green Bank, West Virginia called the U.S. National Radio Quiet Zone, a 13,000 square mile area where most types of electromagnetic radiation are banned.

Environmental Illness comes from anything in the environment, seen and unseen forces all around us. Celebrate that you have this amazing warning system within you, and use it to your advantage to stay out of harms way and to stay well.

Using Quantum Biofeedback helped me identify one of my critical perverse energy issues (ELF, geopathic stress), and it can help anyone to identify perverse energy frequencies that maybe creating stress in their lives. Retraining the Body Electric to better handle this perverse energy stress has proven beneficial to my recovery. **Perverse Energies**, known and unsuspected forces whether recognized by our human senses or not, **are stress** and can harm us.

DEFICIENCY OR EXCESS OF NUTRIENTS: The final major stressor category under **Reduce or Remove the Cause of Disease (the Stressor)** is <u>Deficiency or Excess of Nutrients</u>.

Understanding the power of proper nutrition for my body was critical to my own chemical recovery and it also helped me shed excess weight.

With the advice of my SUPERconscious I began to add more coconut milk and oil into my diet. I started to drink only herbal teas of dandelion, chickory, and tulsi with cinnamon, cloves and other spices.

It started to become clear how my entire day could be destroyed with the wrong food choices. I eventually came to see with the SCIO/EDUCTOR that GMO (genetically modified organism) food was also triggering massive inflammation in my entire body. What I learned about patented GMO seeds would be the same invaluable information I had learned about medicines: <u>if it requires a patent then it did not come from nature</u>. These crops do not exist in nature and in order for a GMO to exist, the hand of man had to be involved.

Farmers who use herbicide tolerant GMO seeds can spray glyphosate throughout the growing season, thereby allowing complete saturation of glyphosate at every stage of plant growth. This chemical deluge is done in an attempt to hold down erosion, but what a steep price to pay as glyphosate is now listed as a probable cancer causing chemical. Even worse for the chemical intolerant individual is the fact that you're slowly sickening yourself with every bite you take.

Another form of GMO seed is the pesticide producing crop.

It's designed to make the stomach of bugs eating this GMO plant to break open and die. What happens to people consuming this food? Well for me and others like me, we too have "gut busting" reactions. This stuff is making people's guts leak and my digestive tract bleed.

Since GMO food is being consumed constantly one may not be able to pin point a connection between their symptoms and the foods they eat. But hear me loud and clear, if you're a multiple chemical sensitive individual, eating food that's been drenched in chemicals is a very bad idea. Therefore, it's of utmost importance that you dedicate yourself to eating 100% organic and chemical free aeroponic food. (See Resources) For some of us, this is a matter of life and death. Some may think I'm being dramatic but if you're deathly allergic to peanuts, you must avoid peanuts at all costs. The same is true for those of us allergic to chemicals. Unfortunately for us, if you're allergic or intolerant to chemicals, this is almost impossible because much of our food supply is saturated in chemicals.

So, I present a challenge to you today. If you have not already begun to do so; I challenge you to eat 100% organic, chemical free aeroponic food, and absolutely no GMO food for three months. If you have MCS or CI, I'm confident that you will feel a difference in your health.

For some people, like small children, the elderly, and chemical sensitives, the reaction to GMO food is quick (and for me painful). For others it maybe a cancer diagnosis in twenty years. Morgelleons disease and other potential nightmares could be on the horizon for an unsuspecting population. For those who are seeking more detailed information about GMO you may want to read Jeffrey Smith's books "Genetic Roulette, The Documented Health Risks of Genetical Engineered Food" or you could watch it in a Video "Genetic Roulette." Mr Smith also has a book titled "Seeds of Deception". I also will be going into much more detail about the truth of GMO foods and the future of chemical free aeroponic food in my next book "Alive Everyday with Tomorrow's Medicine."

It's true... you are what you eat. GMO food, synthetic nutrients, and synthetic supplements are extremely harmful for any individual, but exceptionally harmful for the Multiple Chemical Sensitive (MCS) and Chemical Intolerant (CI) individual.

I also came to understand why most vitamins never worked for me; my body would not absorb synthetic versions of nutrients. All they ever did was create a toxic horror for my liver to process.

Ideally we would have all our nutrients come from quality food, but sometimes we need supplementation of a single nutrient to help the body achieve homeostasis. However, any single nutrient is missing a very valuable piece of the picture: synergy. The essential nutrient can be isolated from a food source and put in a pill, but the energy of that same nutrient working in synergy with the other nutrients consumed within that food, fulfills the nutrient desires of our bodies, as designed by God. Synergy is not happening when you take individual nutrients or synthetic vitamins. Even though I would eat large amounts of fruits and vegetables the SCIO/EDUCTOR was telling me I was starving. I could not seem to eat enough food to make this stress reading of starvation diminish.

One day as I was researching how to eat more fruits and vegetables. I stumbled upon a whole food nutrition in a pill (see Resources) as opposed to a vitamin or nutritional supplement. My interest was also to eat more blue and purple food as these are very high in phyto nutrients. Phyto nutrients are very necessary in helping the body to reduce the oxidation from the cells. The more phyto nutrients in a food the higher the score on the ORAC scale (Chapter 9). The higher on the ORAC scale the more anti-oxidant power a food has. This company had a blend of blue and purple berries in their whole food supplement line up. This bit of information was exciting.

With the use of the Quantum Biofeedback and the therapeutic grade Essential Oils your job now is to eat the best you possibly can and excrete. All the goo the Essential Oils help remove, all the benzene molecules that Professor Nelson's technology has pulled out, all those toxins must be excreted from the bowels, kidney, liver, spleen, skin, endocrine, bone and ears. **Lack of vital nutrients is a stressor but so is too much of a nutrient, or a synthetic nutrient, eat the very best food you can.**

Retraining Organs
Nelsonian Medicine Continued

Now that we've covered all of the stressors under category:
#1) Reduce or Remove the Cause of Disease, let's move on to the subsequent categories under Nelsonian Medicine's Flow of Treatment and Cure:

#2) **Treat the Organs Effected or Diseased**: The beauty of Quantum Biofeedback is the retraining of organs with mild electrical stimulation. The body loves to regenerate, we just need to get out of our own way when it comes to the healing process.

During an advanced quantum training class I sat next to an incognito medical doctor. After two days he turned to me and said, "You know you're not fat?"

I burst out with laughter because it was such an off the wall comment as he'd not spoken more than a grunted "good morning."

Then he asked me "You're swollen, what does this device say you're allergic too?"

This is when I quickly shared with him my toluene allergy and the chemical trauma I had most recently been through. We spent the rest of the week in friendly collaboration as I shared with him my knowledge of Essential Oils and how I'd stayed alive with them until I found the Quantum Biofeedback device. He shared why I needed to address the allergy within my body, pointing out that my lymph, liver and digestive organs were swollen. He pointed out that from the organ chart within the medical software program that I was indeed in need of organ restoration, which is done in the "Whole Organ Restore Program" we had just learned about in our class. Learning this program was vital for overcoming the swelling or shrinking trauma that chemicals create in our organs.

After that class any time any organ was highlighted (SUPERconsciousness choices) in this program to be restored I ran it. Each time I felt a little bit of myself come back online. Each time The "Whole Organ Restore Program" was used to retrain my liver it became softer and less tender. My ears and eyes both improved in function and both stopped being sensitive and painful. Eventually my eyes were not so sensitive to the light and I stopped wearing my sunglasses indoors.

The "Whole Organ Restore Program" has helped me get my digestive system organs back on as well as the endocrine system balanced. I know this program is also helping me return myself back to a new normal of health, whole organs working and functioning properly and communicating within each system perfectly together.

#3) **Unblock the Blockages To Flow of Life**: There are many ways we as individuals can get blocked up. Constipation in our digestion, our mental judgments, and in repeating actions that don't get us the results desired. Once I got my organs to regenerate and the toxic goop detoxed off my receptor sites I began to feel the flow of life!

The spine is a major player for your Body Electric. It's the mega highway of electrical pulses taking you through life. Free flowing energy throughout the nervous system is critical for everything to function properly. Any kink is going to disturb the flow. Have you ever had a lamp or an appliance that had a short in it and you had to jiggle the wire, or do some other trick to get it to work properly? Well that's how your body is if it has a kink or pinch in the nerve flow.

The SCIO/EDUCTOR has a spinal program that's been excellent for me. This program is remarkable at releasing trapped energy in my back. There was a long period of time in my life when I needed to visit a chiropractor twice a week. The raindrop oils helped the horrible neck pain, but they couldn't help the many times I overexerted my back working and would need realigning. The SCIO/EDUCTOR spinal programs stopped the need of bi-weekly spinal adjustments. After a decade of regular Quantum Biofeedback retraining I notice less need for adjustments. However, thanks to Quantum Biofeedback retraining of my spine, it's able to better handle stress, my spine is now healthier and more resilient to life's daily stumbles and I only need to seek chiropractic care for life's big tumbles.

#4) **Reduce Symptoms and All Suffering Naturally**:

My main concerns were:

- Acne
- Apathy
- Blisters on my feet along the edges of where glue was in shoes.
- Brain Fatigue
- Cancer
- Chronic Bronchitis
- Dystonia
- Ear and nose pain, both constantly running.
- Extreme Fatigue
- Eyes sensitive to light, tearing.
- Fungal, Yeast Overgrowth
- Hot and cold sweats, trembling during bowel movements.
- Improper function of digestion.
- Interrupted sleep with night sweats.
- Leaky Gut
- Migraine Headaches
- Mood Swings

- Obesity
- Opportunistic Infections
- Pain in heel and bottoms of feet.
- PMS
- Red dots on my skin.
- Red flush of skin when benzene in environment.
- Skin problems, hot spots, cracking skin, etc.
- Sinus Infections
- Shaking and or tingling in my arms, fingers and toes.
- Sore Throats, Earaches
- Splitting skin on my fingers.
- Sudden loss of consciousness or fainting.
- Sudden Overwhelming Anxiety
- Swelling in upper arms and thighs, tender areas around the lymph areas of my body.
- Swollen, Hot Feet
- Swollen Liver
- Throat Closure
- Weakness

What does your list look like? Many of my passed symptoms have been crossed off my list! I have a new list, with things like slowing down the aging process and encouraging my mind to stay sharp and focused. Even though my diet has greatly improved, I'm still not the ideal weight according to the "charts" however I'm not upset about it. I accept myself for all of me! Acceptance of self is another delightful side effect of wisdom and regular use of these solutions.

#5) **Treat Constitutional and Metabolic Tendencies to Disease Patterns or Habits**: The word Constitutional in this sense is a homeopathic term. I have a brief education and limited experience with homeopathy. With my limited knowledge I use the homeopathic frequencies recommended, generated, and recreated by the SCIO/EDUCTOR device with wonderful results. More proof that getting back to homeostasis is possible even with limited experience and an incomplete education.

In a lecture Professor Nelson was asked what was the goal when he developed the QX technology, I was surprised that Professor Nelson's answer was to find the highest resonance for homeopathic remedies. This piqued my interest to learn at least the basics about homeopathy.

The history of homeopathy actual goes back to Socrates and ancient Greece, when Socrates said "similar cures similar" and later this would enter as the first principal of homeopathic theories by Dr. Samuel Hahneman (1755-1843), a German physician. Dr. Hahneman as a faculty member in Leipzig University in Germany became disillusioned with the medical procedures of his day this included drugs, bleeding and allopathy. In 1796 Dr. Hahneman created an inexpensive safe medicine called Homeopathy. Dr. Hahneman based this medicines on three principles.

Dr. Hahneman's Principles of Homeopathy:

- Like cures Like
- Dilution increases potency
- Disease caused by Miasm

Miasm is a word that means "unhealthy atmosphere." How I understand the word in terms of health is in reference to the blood, if the blood is not healthy then neither will anything else in the body be healthy including an offspring. I'm fascinated by the subject of miasm and see the value of retraining this stress from the blood for better health now and healthier future generations.

Dilution increases potency is at the other end of an Essential Oil, but both work to enhance the healing of your body. An Essential Oil can have a concentration of up to one hundred times stronger than the plant and an homeopathic could be diluted many times that, up to a million.

Professor Nelson has designed and developed the SCIO/EDUCTOR in a way that makes it possible to use your own personal expertise and apply it into the use of the device. Homeopathy is an inexpensive and effective medicine, and although reductionist science poo poos Homeopathy as a valid science, they may in the future be surprised when allopathy finds themselves using homeopathic concepts for the future of pharmaceutical medicine.

For me, using Nelson's and Selye's life works definitely is making *my* life work by getting me back to homeostasis and slowing down aging. It's a wonderful thing as a CI, MCS, EI individual that I'm once again able to move about the benzene world and be alive with Tomorrow's Medicine.

<u>Chapter Twelve</u>

Pain Relief and a Nightlight!

"It is always a blessing when a great and beautiful conception is proven to be in harmony with reality."
~Albert Einstein ~

There are constant reminders in my life that I'm dangerously chemically intolerant. In spite of all my efforts to communicate to a new landlady how imperative it was that my new apartment could not be cleaned with any chemicals or sprayed for bugs, I still ran afoul. She seemed so understanding and promised that she would have no problem with these restrictions. Unfortunately, without my knowledge, her landscaper sprayed the lawn one day. When my skin touched a leaf that had been sprayed I felt an intense pain in my ankle and I collapsed with agony inside my apartment.

As soon as I was able I ran myself on the SCIO/EDUCTOR and it turned out the pain I was experiencing was a result of exposure to a toxin called glyphosate, the main ingredient in the lawn spray the gardener had used! It took several hours of running the detox and pain programs on the SCIO/EDUCTOR for the pain to subside. There was a red mark in the shape of a leaf on my ankle where the pain was most intense. In spite of my SCIO/EDUCTOR sessions I was not able to completely rid myself of that deep tissue reminder of this assault to my body. Although the SCIO/EDUCTOR would relieve the pain and I could sleep, however some random but regular daily movement of my foot would signal a trigger to go off and deep within my foot the internal smoldering pain would return.

A few weeks after this incident a friend invited me to a seminar that I didn't want to go to. My foot and ankle were throbbing and I wanted to put myself on the SCIO/EDUCTOR, not attend a seminar. However, this friend insisted I go. He was adamant that I would like the message about this new quantum tool. Even though my mind and foot were saying no, my intuition was telling me to go and that it would be a pleasant experience.

When I arrived at the seminar the pain in my foot and ankle had intensified into a painful limp. By the time we found seats I was rubbing peppermint oil on my ankle and telling my husband it would be time to go soon.

Paul and Lily Weisbart, the developers, introduced The Quantumwave Laser. Paul explained that he and Lily took low-level laser therapy (LLT), a recognized healing modality, and coupled it with quantum physics and a surprisingly effective healing tool for tomorrow was born!

The Quantumwave Laser is a simple idea: take a low level light (LLLT has been studied for decades) source, in this case a low-level laser (LLT) source and digitally program it with a scalar wave. But what is a scalar wave?

A Scalar Wave is:[1]

- Also called a standing wave.

- Not traveling in a line. It does not move from past to present and therefore is a non linear energy.

- Able to weave and dissolve constantly into the present moment.

- Not following a trajectory or direction making it a more of field.

- What makes up the fabric of the universe.

- What the yogis, mystics, and sages have referred to as prana, chi, universal energy, quantum, scalar energy.

- Capable of activating what yogis, mystics, and sages have done through the ages for regeneration: activation of the subtle quantum field.

- The outer reflection of our DNA.

- Also like the spine's flow of energy, which also moves in a scalar wave fashion.

- Capable of dissolving cell memory due to its nonlinear behavior.

Scalar waves are so important to our well being physiologically and psychologically as earthlings that NASA placed Schumann wave generators within manned space flights.[2] A Schumann wave is a scalar wave. Scalar waves are described as reoccurring longitudinal waves. Sound waves traveling through the atmosphere are an example of longitudinal scalar waves. According to Paul, we're clothed in the essence of light energy and it only makes sense to use energy in the form of laser light to rejuvenate our own bodies and cells.

Now they had my attention, Professor Nelson states in **Promorpheus** that "*any minuscule quantum change in a part of matter will involve the release or absorption of a photon. When an electron absorbs a photon it jumps to a higher quantic state. When it releases the photon it goes to a lower state.*" Professor also states, "*DNA is a receiver and transmitter of laser light.*"[3]

Low level light therapy (LLLT) has been around for decades with volumes of research and (over 3500 studies) supporting the safety and effectiveness of LLLT.[4] LLLT research has shown it enhances healing.[5] Today coupling the low-level laser source (LLT) source and the scalar wave is leading edge technology and over 70 years later, low level light therapy (LLLT) is still not mainstream information.[6] Again we have a safe, simple, and proven effective healing modality that people simply do not know about due to the controlled atmosphere within the health care system of the United

States. Max Plank presented the idea of healing with light in 1899,[7] and veterinarians have been applying it for decades on our pets.

Later I would learn that the low level light therapy (LLLT) is an <u>incoherent</u> light and does not reach the mitochondrial region. The laser diode for the low-level therapy (LLT) is a strong beam of <u>coherent</u> light. Coherent light is effective in stimulating the mitochondrial output of ATP. Coherent light stimulates regeneration by increasing the ATP output (up to 150%), fueling cells and stimulating regeneration.[8]

While I sat and integrated their new information into my cache of quantum knowledge, my glyphosate injured foot and ankle increased throbbing to the point I was squirming in my chair.

When the audience was asked, "Is anyone in pain today?"

I was the first to raise my hand and was invited to be included in the demonstration. We were given an odd hand held tool with dials on one side and what looked like a circle of lights on the other. Our instructions were to place the laser over our adrenals and begin a protocol the developer called "The Unified Field Protocol." Doing as I was told I put this device on my adrenals for a few minutes. My ankle and foot were in so much pain that I finally put the light over those painful areas. At first the throbbing increased for a moment and then released down a little. It would go through this ebb and flow of pain but with each cycle the pain decreased.

After an hour the pain on my ankle and foot had lessened enough that now I was only feeling my old, usual painful areas. One of those areas is my right shoulder. The little tool sat so nicely on my shoulder and after a few minutes the discomfort melted away like butter on hot toast.

I turned to my husband and said, "Somehow we're going home with one of these!"

Stillpoint Now

There was a lot of wonderful energy in the room as we were introduced to the concept of being in a state of rest, being referred to as "Stillpoint." This state of being finds its foundation in the yogic practice of resting in the "space between the breath." The Weisbarts say it best in their book: *"The Stillpoint process is about unwinding and clearing stress, tension, dis-ease, polarity and allowing they body and its systems to reset in the non-linear and Quantumfield state, so that it can then have abundant energy to be used like sunlight for regenerative purposes."*[9]

Scalar waves, as discovered by Nikola Tesla, are naturally occurring neutral waves of earth energy that can be programmed with frequencies that return polarized energy (pain and karma are examples of polarized energy) to neutral[10] bringing the system (like the human body) back to neutral point. This neutral point is what Paul and Lily call "Stillpoint" which can be further explored at their retreats of the same name. (see Resources)

For the first six months of owning the Quantumwave laser, I did it my way. I would play around with different settings and would notice different sensations with each setting. If I was hurt I put it on the "Unwind" setting for a few minutes and then I would put it on "Relief" for pain. Some settings cut through pain and others made me feel relaxed. One setting would wake me up! I decided I wanted to understand this tool better so I could begin sharing it with others.

I attended several Quantumwave laser seminars over the next few years. I learned to surrender to the developer's instructions and began a daily twenty minute session using the "Unified Field Protocol." I began experiencing this tool on a new and different level. After three months of daily "Unified Field Protocol" sessions I felt a large sigh well up within my body and I released this tremendous sound from deep within my inner core.

It was incredible.

That night I slept well for the first time in ages and woke up feeling refreshed. At the next Stillpoint seminar I felt a shift in my experience during the Stillpoint exercises Paul Weisbart lead us through. It felt as if invisible chains fell off my right shoulder and arm. I began to look at this FDA approved tool for pain relief and inflammation in a totally new light.

The Quantumwave laser with it's scalar technology is designed from the perspective of energy and wellness, instead of from a perspective of a medicine and disease. I found that the more I used my laser the more quickly my body responded to resting and clearing the polarity from my Quantumfield.

Additionally, the laser comes with the optional plug in probes to pinpoint the laser wavelength for skin or for denser applications such as bone or inner cell inflammation. These optional probes are available in Red, Infrared and Violet laser diodes giving you three different wavelengths for three different applications to wellness.

Red: is for skin, soft tissue muscle, meridians, and nerves.

Infrared Red: is for bone, tendon, discs, cartilage and brain function. Research studies have shown that Infrared lasers increases the function of brain neurons.[11]

Violet: is a wavelength that is able to hold more information, boosting cell regeneration, immune and neurotransmitter functions. The violet probe has the alchemical information to work on the DNA telomeres, genetic enzymes and stem cells, as well as white matter in lymph and all high spinning ether.

Western medicine, with it's surgery and drugs, excels in trauma recovery and emergency medicine. But what about after the emergency is over? Besides the obvious stress of pain and inflammation of the injured tissue, there are other factors to consider for complete recovery.

The mental body is saying the "why me" and it needs to be heard; the emotional body needs soothing and the spirit needs replenishment.

How Does It Help?

Most people are aware of lasers used in surgery and other cutting and or burning applications. These are called **hot** lasers and require special training and protection. The Quantumwave laser is a **cold, non cutting** laser. Cold lasers are safe[12] and as easy to use as a flashlight.

The safety and effectiveness of using light to heal wounds is well researched and documented.[13] And then there's Professor Nelson's theory of the interaction of light with matter (called Quantum Electro Dynamics), imagine all those photons jumping your electrons up to a higher quantic state! Resulting in reduced inflammation and pain. In a live blood analysis I have seen blood cells that are clumped up with distorted shapes before the "Unwind" protocol. After twelve minutes on the tailbone with "Unwind" the cells become healthy looking and round, white blood cells become more active.

This is a tool that requires little instruction to bring relief and it's very easy to work with. The soft, cold, non cutting laser is a safe and effective tool for everyday use for everybody in the home, including pets.

With the Quantumwave Laser cell memory can be erased.

With the Quantumwave Laser cell memory from injured tissues can be erased. This is very important. Why is this important to the multiple chemical sensitive individual? *"Injured tissue is easier for pathogens to move into and make a home. Injured tissue also makes <u>a good storage place for toxins</u>, especially if far away from the brain and vital organs."* Dr. James R. Overman, ND, author of ***Overcoming Parasites Naturally*** told me this personally when I spoke with him in regards to the rush of movement happening in an area where I had broken a bone years before. Hulda Clark's research into toxicity and cancer found the body[14] is handicapped when parasites flourish especially when the liver is full of pollutants. In her research she found that the most damaging of solvents is benzene; with the runners up being isopropyl alcohol, xylene, wood alcohol, methylene chloride and trichloroethane,[15] which are all an offspring of the mother solvent.

Injured tissue needs help regenerating. Erasing cell memory is of paramount importance in helping the Body Electric recover from all traumas. Although we all commonly believe that sleep begins the healing process, the truth is that sleeping begins the process of the body's cells remembering the injury. Using a combination of healing light, whole food nutrition, plant based medicine, and retraining with quantum technologies erases the cell memory of the traumatized cells. Each day I applied Essential Oils, used the laser over my glyphosate injury. I would place the laser hand unit over the painful area for an hour. I would run 20 minutes on the laser programs:

- Unwind
- Quantum
- Vital

Every few days I ran the SCIO/EDUCTOR programs to detox and repair the injured cells. Over a year of working with all the solutions in this book one day during a session the smoldering pain abruptly stopped. With this and other injuries the solutions brought forth in this book, Essential Oils, the SCIO/EDUCTOR and the Quantumwave Laser have exceeded my expectations, and each has increased the speed at which my healing progressed.

My Incredible Results

My Quantumwave laser side effects:

Side Effect #1 - Less aging of skin. From my personal experience the Integumentary system (the hair, skin, and nails) absorb and store light. If I use my laser and any of the probes on my face, I glow with radiant health.

Side Effect #2 - Nail fungus disappeared on my big toe after I developed the habit of daily use of the laser.

Side Effect #3 - Pain relief without drugs. I find that it's remarkable for pain relief. It was, after all, what made me fall in love.

Side Effect #4 - Inflammation relief. With regular usage I noticed that the inflammation response was easier to process and eliminate.

Side Effect #5 - Erasing cell memory. The Quantumwave Laser has proven to me that I can erase cell memory and my body will regenerate remarkably well if I give it the tools and support it needs.

Learning to erase cell memory is one of the best unexpected consequences I've experienced with following the quantum way of healing. Injured tissue needs relief of inflammation and pain. The Quantumwave Laser's quantum technology is far above average for speeding the healing process.

One of my favorite examples of re-training cell memories involves a decade's old cut on the bottom of my foot. Around age nineteen I had stepped on a broken bottle while running barefoot. It left a nasty gash and eventually healed with an ugly lumpy scar. Occasionally I would feel a pain in that area if I stepped on it wrong, like stepping onto a ladder rung for example. The SCIO/EDUCTOR's message from my SUPERconscious was "toxic scar." When I ran the program for this "toxic scar" the bottom of my foot with the scar would tingle.

Once I introduced the Quantumwave laser to my healing regime the scar on the bottom of my foot would itch. One day it became *very* itchy, red, and swollen. When I rubbed the area it was tender, but if I lightly scratched at it grains of sand would be left on my fingertips. I used all of my tools on that toxic scar and now I can't even see where the mark is!

In working with others, I've observed injuries healing in record time, surgeries avoided, and all without leaving permanent reminders. One brave multiple chemical sensitive (MCS) individual also chose to try all of the solutions I had used for my chemical trauma for a serious injury. Each modality was used daily. Within two weeks all pain and evidence of the injury was gone and full movement had returned. Five years later he has not had any additional problems with the injury.

Light is of vital importance to us in the obvious ways, like not stumbling around in the dark, however in the less obvious ways, like in our tiny cells, we may not notice. Photons are the energy that makes things happen, the garden shows us this with seeds, water, and sunlight. Nelson states it clearly in **_Promorpheus_**; *"DNA is a receiver and transmitter of laser light."*

This brings it all home, healing with light is part of Tomorrow's Medicine.

<u>Chapter Thirteen</u>

The Anti-Steroid

*"We shall require a substantially new manner of thinking
if mankind is to survive."*
~Albert Einstein~

Before I get into my final solution I just want to say that I've been encouraged to leave this chapter out of the book. However, I've refused to follow that advice for quite a few reasons. First, it's important for me to live in integrity and if I removed this part I would be breaking the promise I made to you to share everything that worked for me. Secondly, because it's the most ethereal of the tools for tomorrow. These tools are unfamiliar but that's part of the path that got me back to health. I would be remiss if I didn't share this information with you. How it came to me, what it is, and how it helped me could be a book all by itself. However, for the purposes of this book I will just touch on the high points: How it helped me live with CI and how it may help others with CI, EI, and MCS.

We come to the final tool of the future by going back to the past. It was New Year's Eve, 1981. There was emptiness in my life that was no longer filled by holding my beautiful baby girl. Confused by the year's medical results, remember this is the year when I was diagnosed with PMS, toluene allergy, and spent three days in a coma from lead poisoning. I still was not feeling my normal, energetic self. At the same time I came to the realization that my marriage wasn't what I had fooled myself into believing it to be. At the stroke of midnight I ushered in 1982 alone, drunk, and unhappy.

I found myself on my knees with a soulful prayer asking God, "What's my purpose in life?"

With no answer forthcoming I went to bed. That night I had

the most vivid and real dream I've ever had. It was one of those dreams that stays with you forever. A lucid one in which every detail is clear and intact. When I awoke I was not sure where I was or what day it was, and oddly I did not have a hangover!

The Dream

The Dream began in darkness and my feet were stuck deep into the Earth. Every time I lifted my feet it was a monumental task as the land rose up with the lifted foot. Suddenly, shadowy figures started to chase me. I struggled to lift my feet higher and faster. Panic set in while I attempted to escape the shadow figures. As in the way of dreams, I found myself surrounded by geometric shapes spinning around me. Next appeared round things with holes in the middle. They reminded me of colorful lifesavers. When these colored lifesavers swirled around me I was able to lift my feet freely and run.

As I ran, I neared the edge of a cliff. In the distance there was a far away light piercing the darkness. Without fear I ran off the edge of the cliff towards the pinpoint of light; suddenly there was bright light and I was no longer on my feet! I was soaring free of gravity, free from shadowy figures, free from darkness. I was flying surrounded by spinning clear geometric shapes and multicolored lifesavers.

The Dream didn't answer any immediate issues in my life, but I knew it was extraordinarily important. I spent the next two decades attempting to find the meaning of that vivid mysterious dream. Everyone I shared it with thought it was intriguing but no one, not even a professional dream interpreter could unravel the puzzle with a satisfying answer. Over the years The Dream would run itself through my psyche, full of every detail as if I had just dreamt it. It left me with a sense of wonderment at the riddle I couldn't figure out. The answer would eventually come, but unfortunately it took quite a few health scares to lead me to the information I desperately craved.

A Fibroid Mountain and an Angry Mole

Fast forward to 1999. At this point in my illness journey I was being forced to surrender a large three and a half pound fibroid tumor over to the surgeons and trust that I would get through the anesthesia with the grace of God. I had just been introduced to therapeutic grade Essential Oils. There was no Quantum Biofeedback in my life, and the laser had not yet been developed. I was going to have to step back, have faith, and surrender to this turn of events.

Recovery from the fibroid tumor surgery was not going well for me (although my surgeons were very pleased). Issues with my recovery were increasing every time I was exposed to any chemical in my environment. My abdomen was swelling. I developed a cough. My eyes were very sensitive to the light and I was miserable with internal heat and swelling.

I found myself asking the Universe once again, "Why am I here?"

I would moan through the misery, "Is this all there is to life? Swelling, pain, and drudgery!?"

Surely there's a better way I began to ask... again. Little did I know that an answer was about to be presented into my life, but not before another huge health scare.

In the early fall a scary, angry, brownish red mole had appeared on my right cheek. I consulted my doctor of Chinese medicine who was alarmed by it and wanted me to see a dermatologist. Heather, the friend who introduced me to Essential Oils started bringing me a bottle of water she called "wings water." I would drink the "wings water" daily during a job we worked on together. It looked like regular water in a clean, recycled glass juice bottle. She said it would make my herbal supplements stronger if I took them with the "wings water." The water was also said to help prevent cancer.

I happily drank the water with my regiment of herbal supplements. On the last day of the job, exactly 21 days of drinking "wings water," this potentially dangerous mole fell off into my hand with no mark, scar, or pain. I needed to learn more about this "wings water."

In late October I was invited to attend Heather's "Lightworkers' Cottage" where she was hosting a mini healing seminar on the "wings water."

The seminar was attended by about a dozen people. A few of these people had experienced the "wings water" and like me were excited to learn more. We would learn that the "wings water" was made by placing a small glass tool inside a pitcher of clean filtered water and letting it sit overnight.

That morning I was half listening to the introduction being given by a gentleman named Terry. He was describing his wife Cindy's experience with a man who would appear and reappear in their home. He told us he could see the man but only Cindy could fully converse with him. Cindy shared with us that her journey began in October 1997. This man, appeared before her as a tangible visible form. He spoke directly with her telling her he was an Ascended Master. Cindy said she was a bit surprised by his appearance and asked him his name and he told her it was "Lantos."

I felt comfortable with this woman, she was gentle and sincere. I was not the least bit disturbed by the fact an "Ascended Master" named Lantos was visiting her, after all my favorite ascended masters are Jesus and Buddha. An Ascended Master in my mind has mastered the physical fourth dimensional world and can command it. Appearing and reappearing on different dimensions seems a plausible perk if one can command the physical forth dimension plane of existence. I also understand that Ascended Masters live in the sixth dimension and are our teachers to help guide us to also ascend the physical and come to dwell on the sixth dimension where we can regain a fuller perspective of life.

Lantos began immediately instructing her to get a pen and paper to write down information. This information would eventually become instructions on how to build what Lantos referred to as a "Genesis" device.

This pyramid shaped "Genesis" device would later be verified by an esteemed mathematician to be the same proportions of the Pyramid of Giza. Lantos explained to Cindy that the "Genesis" device would be used for energizing glass and other materials to give light and healing to people and the environment.

After explaining this to us Cindy came out with a suitcase. She set it down and opened it.

There they WERE.

Colorful **lifesavers** and **geometric** shapes.

The Dream!

All the shapes and the colors that were in The Dream from so long ago were staring at me from that suitcase! I crawled past everyone to get a closer look. It felt magical and energizing to finally see those shapes in the physical world. The Dream had come true and I was awestruck, deliriously giddy, and drunk on joy. I always knew my dream came from the highest realms of God consciousness and so did these beautiful glass tools of progress, transformation, and regeneration. We are so blessed to have them available to us once again.

I eagerly shared The Dream with Cindy. She seemed interested and sat with me while the others handled and played with the tools. I wanted to know more about where the tools came from. All Cindy knew at the time was that the tools were returning to Earth after being gone since the time of Atlantis. As the years went by, I learned more and more about these amazing tools from my dream. I want to share with you the knowledge of their existence and how they have helped me, so that you too can choose to benefit from their return back to mankind.

How Does it Help?

Cindy shared that her little daughters would play with the colored wheels by setting them up in a circle. They would sit in the middle of the circle of colored wheels. They would take Cindy's hand and lead her to sit in the circle of colorful wheels. I loved this simple idea, and an example of how easy this technology is to use.

BioGenesis® is a technology, a set of tools. BioGenesis® is not a religion and requires no belief in it to work anymore than a hammer requires a belief in it to work. It's simply a set of tools. Tools have always played a role in mankind's passage or transformation from one age to the next. In the beginning caveman had sticks and stones for tools. Eventually heating the stone and attaching it to the stick, caveman was able to create a passage for mankind into a new age with the invention of the spear and hammer. The creation of new tools took caveman out of The Stone Age into The Bronze Age. It takes releasing old ideas and embracing new ones to be part of the crowd that makes it through any passage of one age to the next.

Daily use of these tools is the most beneficial. Sessions are short; five to ten minutes offers subtle, small benefits that add up over the years.

BioGenesis®, the internet, smart phones... these are just some of the new tools for the Age of Enlightenment, also called the Golden Age of Light. The internet is a technology that we cannot access without a tool like a computer, tablet or smart phone. With the computer we now have access to the ethereal internet. This has been a transformational event for our society. BioGenesis® tools are instrumental to our current passage into the Golden Age of Light.

A BioGenesis® brochure explains it best:

"Throughout the ages God has given us tools and teachings appropriate to our times. As we enter this Golden Age of

Enlightenment, we are once again provided with additional tools.
These tools contain the energy of the Birth of Creation."

All of the BioGenesis® tools look like beautiful glass art objects and have been "trained" with the Light of BioGenesis® and therefore contain the Light of Creation. After sixteen years using BioGenesis® tools and attending seminars and trainings I have come to understand that BioGenesis® is not something one does because the verbal mind understands. It's a tool for your highest good and works on a subtle level that possibly only the SUPERconscious mind will recognize as familiar.

In my humble understanding the terms: "The Light of BioGenesis®", "Birth of Creation", and "The Light of Creation" are all referring to the beginning of the creation of man; to a time when we were all pure, innocent, and unblemished and we knew we were powerful reality creators.

The Tools and MCS, CI, EI, and IEI

All of the many BioGenesis® tools can be used for any number of issues facing mankind, including toxicity and environmental stress. The first tool recommendation is for those suffering from EI. Lantos has instructed that we all need a multi colored BioGenesis® Pyramid in our homes. There are two different pyramids; one is clear and eight sided and the other is four sided and multicolored. Both increase positive energies in the environment which can help people with EI.

When you're plagued with EI, you're tuning in and responding to the environment at a very subtle level and you would benefit greatly from the help of a tool that's doing the exact same thing. Lantos suggests placing a BioGenesis® pyramid in the home or workplace as The BioGenesis® Pyramid begins a subtle correction that restores harmony in the environment. My environmental troubles with EMF's and geopathic stress are much less of an issue for me when I work in the presence of a BioGenesis® Pyramid and within a circle of wheels.

These tools are very beneficial for those who have issues with the environment and chemicals. Our cell's growth patterns are continuously being misdirected, traumatized and harmed by benzene and EMFs. All this subtle disruption coming in from corrupt food, petrochemical based medicine and a polluted environment. Our cells need the appropriate instrument of correction. One thing I learned from my stage hand days was "use the correct tool for the job." These tools are for correcting this misdirection on the subtle bodies as well as your physical body. The tools are easy to use and require only a few simple instructions. There are many tools to chose from and each serves a unique purpose. Here is a list of just some of the tools and what they can do:

BioAmplifier® - For those of us with chemical issues there are several other tools within the BioGenesis® tool box that will be of particular interest for you such as the BioAmplifier. It looks like a glass cylinder cut at an angle. It acts like an amplifier for herbs, people, and objects. It amplifies the effects of the other BioGenesis® tools when used in a BioGenesis® session. It is also beneficial in removing toxins. For me, using the BioAmplifier is helpful when used in a session or alone for removing toxins from the body.

BioOscillator® - For help with environmental issues and chemical issues this beautiful tool looks like a futuristic sword. Lantos told us *"The BioOscillator releases toxins, eliminates the pollutants and impurities, and restores the system to the natural state."* This can be done for both the body and the environment. This tool can clear centuries old trapped negative energy.

Wings of Genesis® - This tool is used to create wings water. Placing a Wings of Genesis in a container overnight and then drinking this water in the morning and the evening benefits the correction of misdirected cell growth. An elegant tool that is difficult to describe as it is not a geometric shape and has a delicate artistic flare about it. Using a Bio Amplifier outside the pitcher near the wings tool will strengthens the energy in the water.This tool does not purify the water. It is safe to consume wings water all day.

Wand of Genesis® - Held in both hands, this tool fills voids in and around the individual. Anxiety, addictions, and prosperity challenges are some examples of voids of energy. Again this tool defies my ability to describe as a geometrical shape. The simplicity of its shape is that of a long slender rectangle, however upon closer inspection it becomes a piece of infinity art.

Flame of Genesis® - A tool that offers the body a return to balance from a variety of distortions such as physical trauma, diseased organs and degenerative diseases. This tool looks like its name, a piece of a flame captured in glass.

The Shield of Genesis® - This tool can be worn or kept near you. It is not worn by children or the elderly, they have their own specific tool. The shield generates a field that surrounds the wearer in an invisible field of protection from negativity and disease. This field offers protection when driving a car. It's a small tool that looks like a small shield.

The Wheels of Genesis® - These are the colored lifesavers of The Dream. There are nine color groups with each color group having a Progress, Transformation and Regeneration wheel making twenty seven wheels each with a specific task. These tools bring harmony and help with pain, help with toxic blood and toxicity in general. These beautiful colors are used within a session to personalize and enhance a specific effect.

My Overall Results

BioGenesis® tools are beautiful. Each year I added a BioGenesis® tool to my kit, it took many years to complete my set. Some of the changes I've noticed since bringing BioGenesis into my life include emotions calming down, clarity over past misunderstandings, old arguments coming to a close, and less confusion in general. Once I began to wear "The Shield of Genesis" I noticed an immediate shift in how others perceived me. They became more understanding of my condition instead of judging and hostile.

Once I had the BioOscillator, which for me is a very prized and desirable tool, I felt a definable shift in depression and constipation. I began to see increasingly positive aspects in my mental and emotional well being after using this tool. I was also able to neutralize impurities faster and I was having fewer toxic headaches.

In 2005, when the special effects chemicals came into my work environment and created that massive benzene oil spill in my body, I grabbed my BioGenesis® tools and would try to work on myself. Unfortunately, I was so sick that I couldn't do much. However, when I was awake I would at least hold my tools, even if I wasn't able to actually work with them.

That summer I attended a BioGenesis® seminar and I asked David Demaray, the spokesman for BioGenesis®,

"Why am I not getting over the chemicals like I always have in the past? Could my tools be broken?"

He reminded me of a message Lantos had given us, "The tools of BioGenesis® work only for your highest good."

David reassured me with a compassionate smile, "You must have a higher good."

Amazingly, a few weeks later I was led to the SCIO/EDUCTOR device and Nelsonian medicine. Then a few years after that, I was introduced to the Quantumwave Laser. Sometimes when things seem lost or the darkness is too thick, there's an answer in the stillness. There's a higher good behind the unknown.

One day from the silence it occurred to me that had BioGenesis® worked as expected in 2005, I would not have sought out other tools. Instead, I would still be working on a movie set. As I shuddered at the memory of the smell of benzene and felt the stress of movie production in my back and neck, that's when I got it! BioGenesis® had always been working in the background of my life even when it seemed it was not working.

The life I live now is so much better for me. I'm doing what I love, I'm healthy, and I'm grateful to be joyfully writing this for you now! BioGenesis® has *always* worked for my highest good and continues to do so today.

I found that giving myself mini sessions on my own picture daily has sped up the release of emotions that were locking me into a victim mentality. We were doing this per instruction of Lantos, he told us *"a picture offers less resistance."* As soon as I put the last tool down from my first session on my picture I felt a "zipper" like feeling unzip down the middle of my body from my bottom lip all the way down to my navel. From out of this invisible "opening" came a rush of tears and sobs. For about five minutes I released a deep, soulful cry of anguish and hurt, and then like that it was vanquished by gently rolling waves of love. I felt cleared of victim mentality and had a new clarity about a personal future.

From the beginning Lantos has said *"All will be called to the Light of BioGenesis but few will see the value."* The value here for me is the understanding that I'm indeed a powerful creator of my reality, and with some new tools and instruction they have assisted me on my journey to master my life and how I choose to experience it. I am indeed a reflection of a vast and mighty intelligence that I can access naturally, and fully tap into with the right tools, knowledge, and intentions. And dear reader, so are you.

Over the years I've shared BioGenesis® with people. A majority have felt benefits from being with the tools. A few have been in awe, as I was, overwhelmed by the joy of finding them. It has been very few that have not found them at least interesting and beautiful. I have seen how Lord Lantos was correct when he told us that all will be called to the Light of BioGenesis® but few will see the value. You may be one that will see the value. The value of returning to perfection, the value of less outside interference, and the value of being victorious over the physical world. If you would like to gain a more expansive perspective on BioGenesis® and the Light of Creation, I suggest you go to the their website

184

www.BioGenesisGlobal.com. Listen to the past weekly messages from Lantos, view past webinars, and attend a webinar or live event.

The tools of BioGenesis® helped me cope with circumstances that were beyond my control, allowing me to remain calm in the face of opposition and oppression. I now know that it's been the Light of BioGenesis® leading me step by step out of the darkness and into the possibility of living a full life span in spite of being one of the forgotten citizens in a **benzene nation**.

There was a time when I didn't know if I would live to see my children reach adulthood, or my beautiful grandchild flourish. There was a time when I feared for their well being. There was a time when I felt the sadness my parents would feel to lose an adult child before their own lifetimes were complete. During those times I would sit with my BioGenesis® wand (a tool for anxiety) and say affirmations of wellness. If I felt overwhelmed, I would sit in the circle of wheels and tranquility would return. I could feel my nervous system calm down. Eventually those anxiety filled moments melted away with the arrival of each solution and new times began to emerge.

BioGenesis®, came to me first. The results of a prayer answered in a dream. I believe BioGenesis® is a tool for the Age of Light. I'm happy and grateful to be able to share this valuable piece of the formulation of events that led me back to wellness and homeostasis. Answers to our prayers come to us in many ways and forms. When we release our expectations of what we think these answers should be is when the solution can arrive unimpeded into our hearts.

<u>Chapter Fourteen</u>

Travelers on a Less Traveled Road

"Strive not to be a success, but rather to be of value."
~Albert Einstein~

Each one of us travels a unique passage to find our way in life. With courage and a deep desire to survive I found my way by taking the unbeaten path that led me to the road less traveled. This journey brought me to a world full of health, vitality, and youthful aging! My hope is that my experience will be of value to you, as well as inspire and encourage you to take that next *best* step for your health and well being. Early in my journey with Chemical Intolerance two things became crystal clear: we must each seek out our own personal truths in order to survive and we must become travelers taking a different road... a less traveled road.

Looking in the rear view mirror, my personal truths standout like reflective mile markers. My first marker would be the letter "T" one of the initials of a common food additive, toluene. The thief of my life force. This small and subtle letter would turn my innocent wide-eyed gaze at the world into a myopic investigation of every label (as well as a visit to every library and doctor along the way!). Another milestone glowing back at me would be the profound impact of taking small actions: trusting nature, using critical thinking, and following my intuition. These small actions would in retrospect prove to be the impetus behind some of my most remarkable moments in life.

Just when I thought I had figured out my fair share of health problems, my son's terrifying health ordeal would take me on an even greater venture, deeper and deeper down that less traveled road. Armed with mother's love and left with no other avenues to explore, I took my son's tiny hand in mine and bravely plunged into the unknown. This terrifying adventure led us to true healing support via communication with the physical and subtle bodies. Don't be afraid to be a traveler on the road less traveled for it will take you places most people will never go and give you a new quality of life that many can only dream about.

Valuable Lessons from Our Journey

It is within these pages, my first book, that we begin our odyssey together on the road to being *Alive with Tomorrow's Medicine*. We quickly learned for this trip we don't need to go too far to *"fill up our tanks with gas"* because the Mother Solvent's many offerings of benzene and toluene based products show up in every aspect of our lives. We have her offspring in our food, medicines, cosmetics, gas tanks, and throughout our homes and work place.

In this society we have benzene at the tip of our nose and toluene on our finger tips! That would be funny if it weren't so scary. Benzene is a carcinogen. It also destroys our blood, brain, nerves, immune system, and potentially our future generations should we continue on this destructive path. Despite our knowledge of its dangers, it still continues to be used as the mother solvent of almost all organically synthesized products!

Although too many of us are full of benzene and toluene it doesn't make us anything like a car or truck! Leaving behind the idea of applying reductionism to the human body, we can now begin pursuing a wider thought. This new thought about yourself was expanded by the knowledge that you're a Body Electric complete with other subtle bodies. Your verbal mind can now rest and relax as the SUPERconscious mind interfaces with your Body Electric using Nelson's Quantum Biofeedback devices. While others were throwing around theories about quantum healing here was a person actually doing it.

As hurricane winds blew overhead I huddled inside my tiny house, watching my first lecture on the Quantum Electro Dynamic Field. Each new concept brought me clarity and I felt instant love and admiration for the genius of Professor Nelson. I have observed him become the truth of his own personal experience of life in a hermaphrodite body. Experiencing a near fatal kidnapping, his survival would depend on the birth of an inner divine feminine and he became a she, changing her name to Desire Dubounet.

I learned so much about healing myself from Professor Nelson's teachings but ultimately I would learn more about living from Desire's courage. By her example of staying alive against incredible odds and by his example of critical thinking, love of truth, and respect for God; I found a path back to life, back to my authentic self. I'm honored every time I work with the beautiful technology developed by Professor Nelson, and I rejoice as Desire continues to lead us and guide us with Tomorrow's Medicine. The world has only begun to see what Nelsonian Medicine and quantum technology can do for mankind!

Bringing mankind's first medicine, the plant, back to North America is another solution that I'm deeply grateful for. Dr. Gary Young's own personal story of an injury leaving him in a shattered, paralyzed body is a powerful and inspirational journey from immobilization back to wholeness using God's medicine. His work, sacrifice, and dedication to this ancient art brings us back to the fundamentals of healing. With this solution we begin a new relationship with the power of concentrated plant medication via therapeutic grade Essential Oils.

Gary and Mary Young of Young Living Essential Oils have invested in pristine land and farms, expanding responsible land stewardship around the world. Every year the offerings of Mother Earth's plants increases with more research and discoveries. The Amazon Rainforest has just begun to reveal remarkable healing plants that offer unprecedented therapeutic plant based medicine. We now understand the remarkable power of the essential oils of plants: a molecular match that's just the right size for our human cell's receptor sites!

We've also explored that photons of coherent and incoherent light are all around us, but it's the coherent light, like that of the Quantumwave Laser, that's required for the processing of energy in our cell's ATP factory: the mitochondria. Within this continued expansion of knowledge we're now aware of cellular actions within our atoms moving into higher and lower energy states by absorbing and releasing photons from their covalent bonds our body's own inner starry night sky!

Using the Quantumwave Laser on pain and inflammation has paid rich rewards for me because pain management without chemicals is now easier to achieve. Paul and Lily Weisbart continue to take their message of Still Point, Lasers, and Quantum Energy around the world; developing more tools for the polarity in our environment and other ways to help people live easier with inflammation and pain. This is amazing news for the chemical intolerant individual!

Finally, we arrive to the biggest truth regarding our existence. This tidbit of news is that we're spirit living inside a physical body, emanating energy via our thoughts and feelings into our Quantum Electro Dynamic Field and out onto our shared environment. With the tools of BioGenesis we can direct and shape this energy, remembering that with focused intentions we are powerful reality creators. It's our fundamental truth.

David Demaray, the spokesman for BioGenesis, travels the world bringing the truth and knowledge of BioGenesis. The Demaray family tirelessly strives to establish the golden network of light around our beautiful Earth. Every few years new tools have been added for humanity and the planet. This is one of the most noble causes for light I have witnessed and I'm honored to be a participant. BioGenesis has given us tools to help pierce through the darkness of lies and distortion and is ready to launch us into the next golden age of truth, health, and knowledge.

The Golden Age

You must look very close to find the little bits of evidence in the physical world that there is indeed a Golden Age upon us. One of those clues presented itself in February of 2015 when CVS

Pharmacies announced they would stop selling cigarettes by October. Another hint was the minor victory when the DARK Act was slowed in the Senate, a glimmer of hope for America's food supply. The information in this book is another first ray of the Golden Age. Today, the first day of spring in 2016, I see the same mainstream news empty of truth and incomplete in information and it's down right shocking.

Over the last few decades, I've gone well past shocked and into full out red alert when my research led me to an actual admission from a Monsanto employee.[1] Dr. William Moar, publicly stated that Monsanto had "an *entire department* dedicated to *debunking* anyone who would dare disagree with Monsanto's science." This may explain Dr. Pusztai's experience, a top food scientist who was fired and discredited three days after going public with his findings and concerns regarding GMO food.[2] My intuition again urged me to look deeper, to go past the obvious greed motives, to stop looking for missing science, and instead arm myself with information that can be substantiated. When you look at the serious facts, it's quite disturbing. There's not much that's more serious than dead people. As far as conspiracy theories go most are easy to debunk, but I find it hard to ignore the fact there's a growing list of dead microbiologists and alternative doctors meeting with dastardly and untimely deaths.[3]

It's now apparent that bringing forth the truth takes tremendous fortitude and courage. That's why I'm so deeply passionate about tomorrow's medicine and I hold such profound gratitude for the work and commitment of my aforementioned mentors: Professor William Nelson, a.k.a. Desire Dubounet, Paul and Lily Weisbart, Gary and Mary Young, and The Demaray Family. They have all displayed tremendous courage, self sacrifice, and personal risk in order to bring forth these tools of tomorrow. That's why they're heroes. Each one has contributed a ray of light into a darkly tinted world, with every intention to bring us closer to a Golden Age of Health and Truth; even when it goes against the beliefs of current day thought.

Information and research around these modalities has not

been supported by the mainstream media, medical, and science communities in the United States. However, I have been told that the SCIO/EDUCTOR is being used in hospitals in countries around the world, such as Spain and Hungary. In the U.S., funding for medical research at the university level comes from pharmaceutical big money and the desire for *patentable* benzene based medicine. Therefore it only makes sense that these and other forms of "tomorrow's medicine" are not being researched and brought forth into the medical world.

In the United States, as the world rejects GMO food, biotechnology companies like Monsanto have their lobbyists working against the Delaney Clause, attempting to ram an anti labeling initiative down America's throat. The Delaney Clause is a provision within the 1962 amendment that clearly states: *"No chemical food additive found to induce cancer in man, or after tests, found to induce cancer in animals would be allowed."* Not only will this continue to erode American's right to know what we're consuming in our food... it's also blatantly breaking the law!

As of March 2015, The IARC has released their findings: glyphosate is a *probable carcinogen.* But these patented GMO seed crops flourish in a bath of glyphosate and the GMO initiative continues to push their anti labeling agenda and propaganda, putting profits over the public's health. My heart breaks as I continue to reach out to our elected representatives to protect our rights and they choose big business interests over the welfare of the people or simply don't show up to vote. GMO labeling loses ground without action from those we've elected to protect us. In my mind this is further evidence of ignorance at best and corruption at worst.

Chemical vapors zig zag giant tic tac toe plumes all across the sky showering us with a myriad of chemical offspring from the mother solvent. This overhead assault on the Body Electric creates blockages in the Quantum Electro Dynamic Field. I believe it's the saturation of the mother solvent benzene in our body's endocrine system, disrupting our body electric and destroying our cell's receptor sites that is slowing killing us as a species.

Then there's the pictures flashing across our TV screens of haunted spree killers with vacant eyes, blankly staring at the camera after another massacre, disconnected from themselves. Why is this so rampant? Could it be from low frequencies disrupting normal thought processes? Are prescription psychiatric drugs like anti-depressants suspending the mind in a nightmare state? Traumatized brains pick up on environmental toxins much easier and they disrupt the thought process, increasing the likelihood of "brains gone bad". Time and time again we learn that another shooter was on antidepressant medication and yet so many people shrug their shoulders in apathy and continue to take the pills. What's really going on here?

On page twenty five I wrote, *"Anyone this far in their search for relief deserves to know the whole truth."* Here is some more truth: The pineal gland is our third eye, our connection to our intuition. The pineal gland can become toxic, hardened, or calcified due to chemical and heavy metal poisoning. Benzene, chlorine and fluoride leave our third eyes essentially blind and unable to view what it was designed to see! In this case we lose sight of our intuitive connection. That connection to the source, to the truth of who we really are, creators of our individual life experiences and not what we've become... victims of our own free will, falling into traps of ignorance.

These reasons and a few more are why I'm releasing this book now, before I'm perfect, before this book is perfect. **You deserve to know you have a choice.** Those who are sick deserve a chance to take back their health. Some of us have been ridiculed; fooled and bullied into believing we're lesser citizens because we can't be in the environment, or because our bodies are sick with swollen and distorted organs.

We are not less than people, we are the people that show instant proof of the madness of benzene and EMFs. Before your brain becomes too dull and befuddled from the various poisons in our society... seek out the truth for yourself. With knowledge, courage, and a little bit of gumption you can take back your right to good health and once again be in control of your life. I know this to be true because I have walked this path. I have survived and thankfully, I have made it out alive. I know how hard it is to live with chemical intolerance in a world coated in benzene... and because of that I'm happy and eager to share my solutions so that others may also be happy and healthy again.

I have shared with you my solutions, what I call tomorrow's medicine. I have explained how each one helped me return back to life. For those who would like to know more about integrating this information into your daily life, or if you would like to share this information with someone who is not sick and would like to stay that way, they may find interest in my next book, *Alive Everyday with Tomorrow's Medicine*. The same solutions are shared but with more of an emphasis on everyday issues and will also include other people's experiences with Tomorrow's Medicine.

With the quantum way we can all become well and have a better chance of staying well. We can slow aging and create stronger, healthier future generations without the need for benzene.

But we will need to work together.

You must participate. The Golden Age is here. Do you want to be sick and tired or would you prefer to feel vibrant and glowing with good health? The choice is yours but you must have an intense desire to be alive and healthy; so much of a desire that you're willing and able to open up to new possibilities.

With my blazed trail may others be inspired to find their personal proof that vitality can again be attained... even if one is deathly ill. Through self awareness, critical thinking, optimum life style changes, Nelsonian Medicine, the SCIO/EDUCTOR Quantum Biofeedback devices, Essential Oils, the Quantumwave Laser, and BioGenesis® a new quality of life was possible for me!

And it can be possible for you... now that you know how to find your way out of the darkness and into *Tomorrow's Medicine*.

Do you feeling like you need to do something but don't know exactly what that is? You could start with the next section of this book; Part Four Resources. Or until your intuition calls you to take your own action, you may desire to use these suggestions as a guideline.

1. **Protect yourself:** In order to protect yourself, you MUST be brave. Brave enough to stand up for your health. When someone is poisoning you, inform them why you don't want to hug them, come to their home, or eat their food. Do not allow yourself to feel embarrassed or bullied into thinking you're over reacting. Tell others when you're feeling the effects of their chemicals. Do not let anyone tell you that you're crazy or a hypochondriac. Remove yourself from these types of relationships or limit your interaction with those who do not respect your health. Being around these type of people is too dangerous for you; its just not worth risking a decline in health. *When we all begin to stand up for ourselves, more and more people will learn to accept and respect chemically intolerant individuals.*

2. **Be well informed:** Know yourself. Know your triggers. Document your symptoms. Share this information with your health care providers. Do your own research.

3. **Speak up:** Request these alternative solutions be prescribed and written up as a prescription. Sure, some doctors may snicker in arrogance, or even become angry, but if they begin to hear it enough, eventually one day they might actually listen. One such doctor listened and prescribed SCIO sessions for a breast cancer survivor and indeed the insurance company purchased the device and paid for the Quantum Biofeedback Specialist to run this device. But it took a doctor with compassion and courage to look beyond the basics of today's medicine and be open minded enough to try a different way. It takes a special kind of doctor, one who still has some degree of critical thinking; a medical doctor who is not resistant to the idea that "quality of life" over "standard of care" is a priority.

Grassroots action by us, in our doctor's offices is one way we can work together to change the mainstream thoughts of drug based medicine into a true alternative health care covered by mainstream insurance companies. I know it's hard, doctors are limited in time with each patient, but make the most of your ten minutes and ask for a written prescription for Quantum Biofeedback and specifically the devices discussed in this book, otherwise you may be sent 1970's equipment.

4. **Speak up even louder!:** No longer remain silent, speak to all who are saturated in benzene. Watch how your local elected officials vote and then call them if they're supporting polluted politics with special interests. The good guys are interested in your opinion, and the ones involved in special interests need to be watched. You will feel more empowered if you take this action. After all, it's your basic right as an American to peacefully express your opinion. We are here to respect Earth and save others from the destruction of boiled benzene, but only when we stand up for ourselves, can we begin to save others.

5. **Read labels:** Look up words you don't know. Your life depends on it! Demand clean food, clean beauty products, and plant based cleaning products by not purchasing the chemical crap. Then call the companies and tell them exactly why you're not buying their products anymore.

6. **Love yourself:** You are special. There is no one in the world like you. You are a divine individual. You deserve to be healthy and happy. Love yourself like your life depends on it... *because it does.*

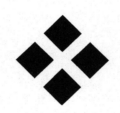

PART FOUR:

The Resources

This section is dedicated to products, information and services that help me stay well. As time brings progress, I invite you to check for updated products and information on:

➢ http://www.alivewithtomorrowsmedicine.com
➢ http://twitter.com/kristymooreher1
➢ https://www.facebook.com/tomorrowsmedicine/

<u>Chapter Fifteen</u>

MSDS: Material Safety Data Sheets

"Everyone who is in the business of dispensing reliable information today has the duty to enlighten the public. For even a conscientious person cannot reach reasonable political conclusions without trustworthy, factual information."
~Albert Einstein~

Being chemically aware includes knowing every ingredient and components of ingredients of what is in everything you put in you and around you. Going to the source of information on each chemical is a good place to start.

My experience with any MSDS has been that it shows a variety of information that changes from sheet to sheet and year to year. I have compiled the findings from several MSDS sources on the basic ingredients found in many everyday products available today. These are all now found easily online. One source I used was National Institute for Occupational Safety and Health or NIOSH's Guide to Chemical Hazards http://www.cdc.gov/niosh/npg/npg.html Another information source is the U.S. National Library of Medicine's Toxnet, www.toxnet.nlm.nih.gov/cgi-bin/sis/search2 a toxicology data network. These MSDS are here to help you learn how serious these chemicals are, even if you are not sensitive and not intolerant. As you dig deeper into the names of every chemical in your food, beauty care, cleaning care and medical care, your inner benzene becomes more apparent. Of all that you put on and in yourself, how much is organically synthesized using the Mother Solvent and her offspring?

Safety Data sheets are organized into distinct sections. For our purposes in this book we will focus on the toxicology and health information. This section can also be full of acronyms and abbreviations that you may not be familiar with.

Agency Acronyms

Agencies that release facts on benzene and toluene:

ACGIH: American Conference of Governmental Industrial Hygienist

ATSDR: Agency for Toxic Substance and Disease Registry

CDC: Centers for Disease Control

DHHS: U.S. Department of Health and Human Services

EPA: Environmental Protection Agency

FDA: Federal Drug Administration

IARC: International Agency for Research on Cancer

NTP: U.S Department of Toxicology Program

NIOSH: National Institute for Occupational Safety and Health

OSHA: Occupational Safety & Health Administration

Health Hazard Labels

Chemicals each have a Health Hazard Label to inform of the level of hazard the chemical has on humans. The system is numbered with the following designations:

Health Hazard Labels:

0- No significant risk
1- Irritation or minor injury
2- Temporary or minor injury
3- Major injury likely
4- Life threatening, major or permanent damage may
   result from a single exposure

The terms used to designate the injury or permanent damage are:

CARCINOGENIC: A substance that has the potential to cause cancer.

EMBROTOXIC: A substance toxic to human embryo.

FETOTOXIC: A substance toxic to animal fetus, toxic to human fetus.

MUTAGENIC: An agent such as chemical or radiation that increase mutation.

TERATIGENIC: A substance or agent that can interfere with normal embryonic development.

TERATOGENIC: A substance or agent that is capable of interfering with normal embryonic development causing birth defects.

Studies are conducted to evaluate the lethal dosage for humans, these results are complied from laboratory animal testing and used as a guideline for humans. (I find this aspect disturbing and feel that if we just used plant based substances there would be no need for cruel animal testings and any of the following terms!)

LD50 Lethal Dose Fifty: the dose of the substance expected to cause death of 50% of the experimental animal population.

LC50 Lethal Concentration: the concentration of the substance in air, and expected time to cause death in 50% of the experimental animal population.

LDL Lethal Dose Low substance introduced by any route but inhalation to have caused death in humans and animals

LCL Lethal concentration of substance introduced by inhalation reported to have caused death in human or animals.

TDL Toxic Dose Low of substance to which humans or animals have been exposed and reported to produce a toxic effect other than cancer.

<u>TOLUENE</u>

Notes: Synonym:
Toluol, Tolu-Sol; Methyl-benzene, Methacide: Phenylmethane, Methylbenzol

Class 1B Flammable Liquid[1]

Health Hazard: 2

POTENTIAL ACUTE HEALTH EFFECTS:
Hazardous in case of skin contact (irritant), of eye contact (irritant), of ingestion. of inhalation. Slightly hazardous in case of skin contact (permeator[3]).

POTENTIAL CHRONIC HEALTH EFFECTS:
The substance may be toxic to blood, kidneys, the nervous system, liver, brain, central nervous system (CNS). Repeated or prolonged exposure to the substance can produce target organs damage.

CARCINOGENIC EFFECT:

A4 (Not classifiable for human or animal) by ACGH,

3 (Not classifiable for human.) by IARC.

TERATIGENIC: Not available

MUTAGENIC EFFECTS: Not available

DEVELOPEMNTAL TOXICITY : Not Available

TOXICOLOLGICAL INFORMATION:

Routes of entry through skin, Dermal contact. Eye contact. Inhalation. Ingestion.

Toxicity to Animals:

Warning the LC50 VALUES ARE ESTIMATED ON THE BASIS OF A 4-HOUR EXPOSURE. Acute oral toxicity (LD50), 636mg/kg (Rat), Acute dermal toxicity (LD50) 14100mg/kg (Rabbit). Acute toxicity of the vapor (LD50) 440mg/kg hours (Mouse)

Chronic Effects on Humans:

CARCINOGENIC EFFECTS:

A4 (Not classifiable for human) by ACGIH, 3 (Not classifiable for human.) by IARC

May cause damage to the following organs: blood, kidneys, the nervous system, liver, brain, central nervous system (CNS).

Other Toxic Effects on Humans:

Hazardous in case of skin contact (irritant), of ingestion, of inhalation. Slightly hazardous in case of skin contact (permeator).

Special Remarks on Toxicity to Animals:

Lowest Published Lethal Dose: LDL (Human)- route: Oral; Dose 50 mg/kg LDL (Rabbit)- Route: Inhalation: Dose 55000ppm/40min

Special Remarks on other Chronic Effects on Humans:

Detected in maternal milk in human. Passes through the placental barrier in human. Embrotoxic (toxic to embryo) and /or fetotoxic (toxic to fetus) in animal. May cause adverse reproductive effects and birth defects (teratogenic). May affect genetic material (mutagenic).

Special Remarks on Other Toxic Effects on Humans:

Acute Inhalation:

Inhalation Health Effects:

Skin:

Causes mild to moderate skin irritation. It can be absorbed to some extent through the skin.

Eyes:

Causes mild to moderate eye irritation with a burning sensation. Splash contact with eyes also causes conjunctivitis, blepharospasm, corneal edema, corneal, abrasions. This is usually resolved in 2 days.

Inhalation:

Inhalation of vapor may cause respiratory tract irritation causing coughing and wheezing, nasal discharge. Inhalation of high concentration may affect behavior and cause central nervous system effects characterized by nausea, headache, dizziness, tremors, restlessness, lightheartedness, exhilaration, memory loss, insomnia, impaired reaction time, drowsiness, ataxia, hallucination, somnolence, muscle contraction or spasticity, unconsciousness and coma. Inhalation of high concentration of vapor may also affect the cardiovascular system (rapid heartbeat, heart palpitations, increased or decreased blood pressure, dysrhythmia), respiration (acute pulmonary edema, respiratory depression, apnea, asphyxia), cause vision disturbances and dilated pupils, and cause loss of appetite.

Ingestion:

Aspiration of Toluene into the lungs may cause chemical pneumonitis. May cause irritation of digestive tract with nausea, vomiting, pain. May have effects similar to that of acute inhalation.

Chronic Potential Health Effects:

Inhalation and Ingestion:

Prolonged or repeated exposure via inhalation may cause central nervous system and cardiovascular symptoms similar to that of acute inhalation and ingestion as well liver damage/failure, kidney damage/failure (with hematuria, proteinuria, oliguria, renal tubular acidosis), brain damage, weight loss, blood (pigmented or nucleated red blood cells, changes in white blood cell count), bone marrow changes, electrolyte imbalances (hypokalemia, hypophosphatemia) sever, muscle weakness and Rhabdomyolysis.

Skin:

Repeated or prolonged skin contact may cause defatting dermatitis.

BENZENE

Notes: Also called Naphta

Health Hazard: 2

POTENTIAL HEALTH EFFECTS:
Very hazardous in case of eye contact (irritant), of inhalation. Hazardous in case of skin contact (irritant, permeator), of ingestion. Inflammation of the eye is characterized by redness, watering, and itching.

CARCINOGENIC EFFECTS:
Classified A-1 (confirmed for human) by IARC. 1 (Proven for human.) by IARC.

MUTAGENIC EFFECTS:
Classified POSSIBLE for human. Mutagenic for mammalian somatic cells. Mutagenic for bacteria and/or yeast.

TERATOGENIC EFFECTS: Not available.

DEVELOPMENT TOXICITY:
Classified Reproductive system /toxin /female (POSSIBLE). The substance is toxic to blood, bone marrow, central nervous system (CNS). The substance may be toxic to liver, urinary system. Repeated or prolonged exposure to the substance can produce target organ damage.

TOXICOLOGICAL INFORMATION:
Toxicity to Animals: basis of four hour exposure. Acute Oral toxicity (LD50):930mg/kg (Rat).Acute dermal toxicity (LD50)>9400 mg/kg (rabbit). Acute toxicity of the vapor (LC50): 100007 hours (Rat).

Chronic Effects on Humans:
> Other Toxic Effects on Humans: Very hazardous in case of inhalation. Hazardous in case of skin contact (irritant, permeator), of ingestion.

Special Remarks on Chronic Effects on Humans:
> May cause adverse reproductive effects (female fertility, Embryotoxic and /or fetotoxic in animal) and birth defects. May affect genetic material (mutagenic). May cause cancer (tumorigenic, leukemia) Human: passes the placental barrier, detected in maternal milk.

Special Remarks on other Toxic Effects on Humans:

Acute Potential Health Effects:
> Skin: Causes skin irritation. It can be absorbed through intact skin and affect the liver, blood, metabolism, and urinary system.

Eyes: Causes eye irritation.

Inhalation:
> Causes respiratory tract skin and mucus membrane irritation. Can be absorbed through the lungs. May affect behavior/Central and Peripheral nervous systems (somnolence, muscle weakness, general anesthetic and other symptoms similar to ingestion). gastrointestinal tract (nausea), blood metabolism, urinary tract system.

Ingestion:
> May be harmful if swallowed. May cause gastrointestinal tract irritation including vomiting. May affect behavior/Central and Peripheral nervous systems (convulsions, seizures, tremor, irritability, initial CNS stimulation followed by depression, loss of coordination, dizziness, headache, weakness, pallor, flushing) respiration (breathlessness and chest constriction), cardiovascular system,

(shallow/rapid pulse), and blood.

DIETHANOLAMINE

Notes:

Acronym: DEA. Also listed as Cocamide DEA, Cocamide DEA, Coamide DEA, Cocamide MEA, DEA-Cetyl Phosphate, DEA Oleth-3 Phosphate, Lauramide DEA, Linoleamide MEA, Myristamide DEA, Oleamide DEA, Stearamide MEA,TEA-Lauryl Sulfate, Triethanolamine

Health Hazard:

1 on older MSDS but lately has been 3

POTENTIAL ACUTE HEALTH EFFECTS:

Extremely hazardous in case of skin contact (irritant), of eye contact (irritant), of ingestion, of inhalation. Very hazardous in case of skin contact (permeator). Inflammation of the eye is characterized by redness, watering, and itching. Skin inflammation is characterized by itching, scaling, reddening, or, occasionally blistering.

POTENTIAL CHRONIC HEALTH EFFECTS:

Extremely hazardous in case of skin contact (irritant), of eye contact (irritant), of ingestion, of inhalation. Very hazardous in case of skin contact (permeator).

CARCINOGENIC EFFECTS: Not available.

TERATIGENIC EFFECTS: Not available.

MUTAGENIC EFFECTS: Not available.

Developmental Effects: Not available.

Toxicity:

Not available. Repeated or prolonged inhalation of dust may lead to chronic respiratory irritation.

CARCINOGENIC EFFECT: Not available.

DEVELOPEMENTAL TOXICITY: Not available.

TOXICOLOLGICAL INFORMATION:

Routes of Entry:
Dermal contact. Eye Contact. Inhalation. Ingestion.

Toxicity to Animals:
Acute oral toxicity (LD50):710mg/kg (rat). Acute dermal toxicity (LD50): 12200mg/kg (Rabbit)

Chronic Effects on Humans: Not available.

Other Toxic Effects on Humans: Not available.

Special Remarks on Chronic Effects on Humans: Not available.

Special Remarks on other Toxic Effects on Humans: Not available

SODIUM LAURYL SULFATE

Notes:
Synonym: Sodium dodecyl sulfate Chemical name: sulfuric acid, monododecyl ester, sodium salt

Health Hazard: 2

POTENTIAL ACUTE HEALTH EFFECTS:
Hazardous in case of skin contact (irritant) of eye contact (irritant) of ingestion, of inhalation. Slightly

hazardous in case of skin contact (sensitizer) Severe over-exposure can result in death.

POTENTIAL CHRONIC HEALTH EFFECTS:
Slightly hazardous in case of skin contact (sensitizer).

CARCINOGENIC EFFECTS:
NOT AVAILABLE. Mutagenic Effects: Mutagenic for bacteria and/or yeast.

Teratogenic Effects: Not available.

Developmental Effects:
Not available. The substance may be toxic to skin. Repeated or prolonged exposure to the substance can produce target organ damage. Repeated exposure to a highly toxic material may produce general deterioration of health by an accumulation in one or many human organs.

DEVELOPEMNTAL TOXICITY: Not Available

TOXICOLOLGICAL INFORMATION:

Routes of Entry: Inhalation, Ingestion

Toxicity to Animals:
Basis of four hour exposure. Acute oral toxicity (LD50) 1288mg/kg (Rat). Acute toxicity of the dust (LC50)>3900mg/m 1 hour (Rat)

Special Remarks on Toxicity to Animals:
Lowest published Lethal Dose: LDL (Rabbit): Route skin. Dose: 10000 mg/kg

Chronic Effects on Humans:
MUTAGENEIC EFFECTS: mutagenic for bacteria and or yeast. May cause damage to the following

organs: skin

Other Toxic Effects on Humans:

Hazardous in case of skin contact (irritant), of ingestion, of inhalation. Slightly hazardous in case of skin contact (sensitizer).

Special Remarks on Chronic Effects on Humans:

May cause adverse reproductive effects based on animal test data. No human data found.

Special Remarks on other Toxic Effects on Humans:

Acute potential Health Effects:

Skin:Causes mild to moderate skin irritation. May cause allergic reaction (dermatitis).

Eyes:

Causes moderate eye irritation. Inhalation: Material is irritating to mucous membranes and upper respiratory tract. May cause allergic respiratory reaction.

Ingestion:

Causes gastrointestinal tract irritation with nausea, vomiting, hyper-motility, diarrhea, and bloating. May also affect behavior (ataxia, somnolence), and cardiovascular system.

Chronic Potential Health Effects:

Skin:

Prolonged or repeated skin contact may cause allergic dermatitis.

Inhalation:

Prolonged or repeated inhalation may cause allergic respiratory reaction (asthma).

Ingestion:

Prolonged or repeated ingestion may affect the liver.

PROPYLENE GLYCOL

Health Hazard: 1

POTENTIAL HEALTH EFFECTS:
Hazardous in case of ingestion, Slightly hazardous in case of skin contact (irritant, permeator) of eye (irritant) of inhalation

POTENTIAL CHRONIC HEALTH EFFECTS:
Slightly hazardous in case of skin contact (sensitizer)

CARCINOGENIC EFFECT: Not Available

DEVELOPEMNTAL TOXICITY:
Not Available. The substance may be toxic to central nervous system (CNC). Repeated or prolonged exposure to the substance can produce target organs damage.

TOXICOLOLGICAL INFORMATION:
Absorbed thru the skin. Eye Contact.

Toxicity to Animals:
Acute oral toxicity (LD50); 18500 mg/kg (Rabbit). Acute dermal toxicity (LD50)): 20800 mg/kg (Rabbit)

Chronic Effects on Humans:
May cause damage to the following organs: central nervous system (CNS).

Other Toxic Effects on Humans:
Hazardous in case of ingestion. Slightly hazardous in case of skin contact (irritant, permeator), of inhalation.

Special Remarks on Chronic Effects on Humans:
May affect genetic material (mutagenic). May cause adverse reproductive effects and birth defects (teratogenic) based on animal test data.

Special Remarks on other Toxic Effects on Humans:

Acute Potential Health Effects:
May cause mild skin irritation. It may be absorbed through the skin and cause systemic effects similar to those of ingestion.

Eyes:
May cause mild eye irritation. With some immediate transitory stinging, lacrimation, blepharospasm, and mild transient hyperemia conjunctival. There is no residual discomfort or injury once this washed away.

Inhalation:
May cause respiratory tract irritation.

Ingestion:
It may cause gastrointestinal tract irritation. It may affect behavior/central nervous system (CNS) depression, general anesthetic, convulsions, seizures, somnolence, stupor, muscle contraction or spasticity, coma), brain (changes in surface EEG), metabolism, blood (Intravascular hemolysis, white blood cells-decreased neutrophil function), respiration (respiratory stimulation, chronic pulmonary edema, cyanosis) cardiovascular system (hypotension, bradycardia, arrhythmias, cardiac arrest) endocrine system (hypoglycemia) urinary system and Liver, Kidneys

Chronic Potential Health effects.:
Prolonged or repeated skin contact may cause allergic contact dermatitis. Ingestion: Prolonged or

repeated ingestion may cause hyperglycemia and may affect behavior/CNS (symptoms similar to ingestion) and spleen.

GLYPHOSATE

Notes: Synonym: Glycine, N-(Phosphonomethyl)-; Glyphosat; Glyphomax; Roundup®

Health Hazard: 2 in New Jersey, 0 in other states.

POTENTIAL HEALTH EFFECTS:
Hazardous in case of ingestion, Slightly hazardous in case of skin contact (irritant, permeator) of eye (irritant) of inhalation

POTENTIAL CHRONIC HEALTH EFFECTS:
Slightly hazardous in case of skin contact (sensitizer)

CARCINOGENIC EFFECT[4]:
Classified 2A: probably carcinogenic to humans by IARC[5]

DEVELOPEMNTAL TOXICITY:
Not Available. The substance may be toxic to central nervous system (CNC). Repeated or prolonged exposure to the substance can produce target organs damage.

TOXICOLOLGICAL INFORMATION[6]:
Absorbed thru the skin. Eye Contact.

Toxicity to Animals: Acute oral toxicity (LD50); 18500 mg/kg (Rabbit). Acute dermal toxicity (LD%)): 20800 mg/kg (Rabbit)

Chronic Effects on Humans: May cause damage to the following organs: central nervous system (CNS).

Other Toxic Effects on Humans:
Hazardous in case of ingestion. Slightly hazardous in case of skin contact(irritant, permeator), of inhalation.

Special Remarks on Chronic Effects on Humans: May affect genetic material (mutagenic). May cause adverse reproductive effects and birth defects (teratogenic) based on animal test data.

Special Remarks on other Toxic Effects on Humans: Acute Potential Health Effects: May cause mild skin irritation. It may be absorbed through the skin and cause systemic effects similar to those of ingestion.

Eyes: May cause mild eye irritation. With some immediate transitory stinging, lacrimation, blepharospasm, and mild transient conjunctival hyperemia. There is no residual discomfort or injury once this washed away.

Inhalation: May cause respiratory tract irritation.

Ingestion: It may cause gastrointestinal tract irritation. It may affect behavior/central nervous system (CNS)depression, general anesthetic, convulsions, seizures, somnolence, stupor, muscle contraction or spasticity, coma), brain (changes in surface EEG), metabolism, blood (Intravascular hemolysis, white blood cells-decreased neutrophil function), respiration (respiratory stimulation, chronic pulmonary edema, cyanosis) cardiovascular system (hypotension, bradycardia, arrhythmias, cardiac arrest) endocrine system (hypoglycemia) urinary system and Liver, Kidneys

Chronic Potential Health effects. Skin: prolonged or

repeated skin contact may cause allergic contact dermatitis. Ingestion: Prolonged or repeated ingestion may cause hyperglycemia and may affect behavior/

Chapter Sixteen

Resources

*"I do not like to state an opinion on a matter
unless I know the precise facts."*
~Albert Einstein~

Beauty Products Database

www.ewg.org/skindeep

BioGenesis

Website: www.BioGenesisGlobal.com
Phone: 888-722-2213

Cleaning House Chemical free

I use Thieves Household Cleaner, white organic vinegar, hydrogen peroxide, and baking soda.

There are more household products made safe with essential oils by Young Living.

www.youngliving.org/kristyhernandez
Thieves Household Cleaner Item #3743
Thieves Fruit and Veggie Soak and Spray Item # 5344
Thieves Laundry Soap Item # 5349
Thieves Dish Soap Item #5350

Customized Teas

Good Life to Go:
Organic teas, customized teas
Website: www.goodlifetogo.net/store
also on   www.Amazon.com
Email: inquiries@goodlifetogo.net
Phone: 407-761-7189

Essential Oils

www.youngliving.com/kristyhernandez

Essential Oils	Order Number
Believe	**Item # 4661**
Blue Cypress	Item # 3083
Body Wash	*Item # 3745*
Brain Power	**Item # 3313**
Clove	Item # 3524
Clary Sage	**Item # 3521**
Cedarwood	Item # 3509
Di-Gize	**Item # 3321**
Difusers:	*Item # 3660*
DragonTime	**Item # 3327**
Endoflex	**Item # 3333**
Exodus II	**Item # 3338**
Frankincense	Item # 3548
Fennel	Item # 3542
Geranium	Item # 3554
Hope	**Item # 3357**
Household Cleaner,	
Thieves	*Item # 3743*
Joy	**Item # 3372**
Juva Cleanse	**Item # 3395**
Lady Sclareol	**Item # 3376**
Lavender	Item # 3575
Lemongrass	Item # 3581
Mister	**Item # 3381**
Ocotea	Item # 3556
Oregano	Item # 3605
Panaway 5 ml	**Item # 3391**
Panaway 15 ml	**Item # 3390**
Peace and Calming	**Item # 5327**
Peppermint	Item # 3614
Raindrop Technique	*Item # 3137*
Release	**Item # 3408**
Sacred Frankincense 5 ml	Item # 3550
Sacred Frankincense 15 ml	Item # 3552
SARA	**Item # 3417**

Sage	Item # 3632
Thieves	**Item # 3423**
Transformation	**Item # 3060**
Trauma Life	**Item # 6350**
Toothpaste	*Item # 3039*
White Angelica	**Item # 3428**
Valor	**Item # 3430**
V-6 Carrier Oil	*Item # 3031*
Ylang-Ylang	Item # 3659

GMO Information

Books and Films:

http://responsibletechnology.org

Books by Jeffery M. Smith

Genetic Roulette

Seeds of Deception

Hidden Dangers in Kids Meals

GMO free Shopping Guide:

http://nongmoshoppingguide.com/

Herbs

Organic and wild-crafted herbs

Website: http://www.goodlifetogo.net/store

also on www.Amazon.com

Email: inquiries@goodlifetogo.net

Phone: 407-761-7189

Indoor Garden

Grow your own petrochemical free tower of food.

http://www.kristyhernandez.towergarden.com

Information on Essential Oils

The Center For Aromatherapy Research Website:

http://www.raindroptraining.com/care/yleo.shtml

Chemistry of Essential Oils Made Simple: God's Love Manifest in Molecules by Dr. David Stewart

Healing Oils of the Bible by Dr. David Stewart

Other Books by Dr. Stewart

http://www.amazon.com/David-Stewart/e/B001KCS7FM/ref= dp_byline_cont_pop_book_1

Essential Oils Integrative Medical Guide, Building Immunity, Increasing Longevity, and Enhancing Mental Performance with Therapeutic-Grade Essential Oils by D.Gary Young, N.D.

People's Desk Reference for Essential Oils

Website: www.lifesciencepublishers.com

Current editions are now available online from the publisher as well as in printed hardback books.

Juice Plus+

http://www.kristyhernandez.juiceplus.com

Professional Validation of Claims

World Health Products Ratings Service

http://www.whprs-ratings.com/

The VoltAmetric Cybernetic Loop Technology includes several generations of devices QXCI, EPFX, SCIO, INDIGO, EDUCATOR, and EDUCTOR.

Quantum Biofeedback Session Appointment

305-910-6345

http://www.alivewithtomorrowsmedicine.com

Quantumwave Lasers

Website: http://kristy.ilovemylaser.com

Raindrop Essential Oils

The Raindrop Technique® Essential Oil Collection
Item # 3137
https://www.youngliving.org/kristyhernandez

Raindrop Practitioner Miami and New York

http://www.hands2hearthealing.com

SCIO/EDUCTOR

Purchase device and book Sessions:
305-910-6345
www.alivewithtomorrowsmedicine.com

Tea

Good Life to Go:
Organic customized teas
Website: www.goodlifetogo.net/store
also on   www.Amazon.com
Email: inquiries@goodlifetogo.net
Phone: 407-761-7189

Therapeutic Grade Essential Oils

Young Living Essential Oils Website:
https://www.youngliving.org/kristyhernandez
Email: kristylove@hushmail.com
YLEO Phone: 800-371-3515
Kristy Hernandez, Member#: 313657

Tinctures

Good Life to Go:
Website: www.goodlifetogo.net/store
also on   www.Amazon.com
Email: inquiries@goodlifetogo.net
Phone: 407-761-7189

Whole Food Nutrition: (not the corporate store, but from nature!)

Juice Plus+ :

Thirty fruits and vegetables without the salt and sugar, but keeping enzymes and synergy intact.

www.kristyhernandez.juiceplus.com

MILA:

Milled chia seed with highest available omegas in whole food form.

www.alivewithtomorrowsmedicine.com

MASTER FORMULA:

Young Living Essential Oils now carries a whole food supplement.

www.youngliving.org/kristyhernandez

Master Formula Item #5292

The Professor Keeps on Giving, Access to More Information, Increase Your Awareness, Tell Others

Prof Desire' Dubounet Life Stories
http://www.downloads.imune.net/medicalbooks/DesirePosters/Desire%20Dubounet%20Wikipidia.pdf

http://rationalwiki.org/wiki/William_Nelson

Desiré Dubounet, The Hero Part 1
https://www.youtube.com/watch?v=9A6qOsSBjEU

Desiré Dubounet, The Hero Part 2
https://www.youtube.com/watch?v=ARcBg_OrwHg

Intellect is the final frontier, Story of Desi's Youth
https://www.youtube.com/watch?v=gQ767ldaraY

Acupuncture Needles Become Medical Equipment because of Desiré
http://www.downloads.imune.net/medicalbooks/Acupuncture%20needles%20become%20medica_
http://www.downloads.imune.net/medicalbooks/Acupuncture%20needles%20become%20medical%20equipment%20because%20of%20Desire%27(1).pdf

Big Tobacco the Evil that does not die
http://medicalexposedownloads.com/PDF/Big%20Tobacco%20the%20Evil%20that%20does%20not%20die.pdf

Bush sells America to the Drug Companies
http://medicalexposedownloads.com/PDF/Bush%20sells%20America%20to%20the%20Drug%20Companies.pdf

Cancer Course
http://www.downloads.imune.net/medicalbooks/Cancer%20course.pdf

Charging the Body Electric Battery - VARHOPE by Brad Vee
Jounson
http://medicalexposedownloads.com/PDF/Charging%20the%20Bo
dy%20Electric%20Battery%20-
%20VARHOPE%20by%20Brad%20Vee%20Jounson.pdf

Definition of Natural vs Synthetic, I mean SINthetic
http://medicalexposedownloads.com/PDF/Definition%20of%20Na
tural%20vs%20Synthetic,%20I%20mean%20SINthetic.pdf

Desire' and Myth Busters Prove man walked on the moon
http://www.downloads.imune.net/medicalbooks/Desire%27%20an
d%20Myth%20Busters%20Prove%20man%20walked%20on%20t
he%20moon.pdf

Desire' Author Editor of Vast Natural Medicine Library with non-
drug treatments for most all diseases
http://medicalexposedownloads.com/PDF/Desire'%20Author%20E
ditor%20of%20Vast%20Natural%20Medicine%20Library%20wit
h%20non-
drug%20treatments%20for%20most%20all%20diseases.pdf

Desire Dubounet finds that Bigotry can be weakened by Equal
Economic Education
http://www.downloads.imune.net/medicalbooks/Desire%20Dubou
net%20finds%20that%20Bigotry%20can%20be%20weakened%20
by%20Equal%20Economic%20Education.pdf

Desire' Dubounet has a Sugar Coated Message for the World
http://medicalexposedownloads.com/PDF/Desire%27%20Duboune
t%20has%20a%20Sugar%20Coated%20Message%20for%20the%
20World.pdf

Desire' Dubounet, the famous TV and Movie Star of Hungary
http://medicalexposedownloads.com/PDF/Desire%27%20Duboune
t,%20the%20famous%20TV%20and%20Movie%20Star%20of%2
0Hungary.pdf

Desire' Dubounet's Biography
http://medicalexposedownloads.com/PDF/Desire%27%20Duboune
t%27s%20Biography.pdf

Desire' helps to design WHPRS the first independent consumer
advice agency for Alternative Medical Devices
http://medicalexposedownloads.com/PDF/Desire%27%20helps%2
0to%20design%20WHPRS%20the%20first%20independent%20co
nsumer%20advice%20agency%20for%20Alternative%20Medical
%20Devices.pdf

Desire' looks at the worst health problems
http://www.downloads.imune.net/medicalbooks/Desire%27%20lo
oks%20at%20the%20worst%20health%20problems.pdf

Desire' Dubounet Saves Natural+ Energetic Medicine with
Research + Evidence-Based Validation
http://www.downloads.imune.net/medicalbooks/Desire%e2%80%
99%20Dubounet%20Saves%20Natural+%20Energetic%20Medici
ne%20with%20Research+Evidence-Based%20Validation.pdf

Desiré's Courage to Think with the Big Head Not the Little (Dick)
Head
http://medicalexposedownloads.com/PDF/Desire%e2%80%99s%2
0Courage%20to%20Think%20with%20the%20Big%20Head%20
Not%20the%20Little%20%28Dick%29%20Head.pdf

EVIL BIG OIL--Why should we dig for oil when we can grow it
http://medicalexposedownloads.com/PDF/EVIL%20BIG%20OIL-
Why%20should%20we%20dig%20for%20oil%20when%20we%2
0can%20grow%20it.pdf

Excess Homophobia is caused by latent secret homosexuality
http://medicalexposedownloads.com/PDF/Excess%20Homophobia
%20is%20caused%20by%20latent%20secret%20homosexuality%
281%29.pdf

Foods That Kill - should be banned and must be avoided
http://medicalexposedownloads.com/PDF/Foods%20That%20Kill%20-%20should%20be%20banned%20and%20must%20be%20avoided.pdf

Forget the tech bubble. Its the biotech bubble you should worry about
http://medicalexposedownloads.com/PDF/Forget%20the%20tech%20bubble.%20Its%20the%20biotech%20bubble%20you%20should%20worry%20about.pdf

Freedom of Choice in Medicine
http://medicalexposedownloads.com/PDF/Freedom%20of%20Choice%20in%20Medicine.pdf

Here are the base medical claims registered and validated by the regulators in our clinical evaluation
http://medicalexposedownloads.com/PDF/Here%20are%20the%20base%20medical%20claims%20registered%20and%20validated%20by%20the%20regulators%20in%20our%20clinical%20evaluation.pdf

Hungary Gets Homeopathy because of Professor Desire
http://www.downloads.imune.net/medicalbooks/Hungary%20Gets%20Homeopathy%20because%20of%20Professor%20Desire.pdf

Index

232

Bibliography

*"The important thing is not to stop questioning. Curiosity has its
own reason for existing."*
~Albert Einstein~

Andersen, U.S., *The Greatest Power in the Universe*, Atlantis
University, 1971.

Archives of Environmental Health: An International Journal,
May/June 1999 issue,Vol. 54, No. 3, pp. 147-149. April
2010. Heldref Publications. *Multiple Chemical Sensitivity:
A 1999 Consensus,* Dec 2012, http://www.heldref.org.

Becker, Robert O. and Gary Seldon, *The Body Electric,* William
Morrow and Company, Inc., 1985.

Dubounet, Desire, *The Messenger Angel, The Messages of the
Angel The Science and Philosophy*, Change The World
Productions, 2010.

Calaprice, Alice, Collected and Edited by, *The Ultimate Quotable
Einstein,* Princeton University Press, reprinted 2011.

Campbell, Collin T., PhD. And Campbell, Thomas M. II,
*The China Study, Startling Implications for Diet, Weight
Loss and Long Term Health ,* Benbella Books, 2006

Clayton L. Thomas, MD, M.P.H.
Taber's Cyclopedia Medical Dictionary 14th Edition, F.A.
Davis, 1981.

Clark, Hulda Regehr, *The Cure For All Diseases,* New Century
Press, reprinted 2007.

Clark, Hulda Regehr, *The Cure And Prevention of All Cancers,*
New Century Press, reprinted 2010.

Fox, Frances, *The Gods Speak Dolphin Wisdom Revealed,* Frances Fox, Inc., 2010.

Green, Glenda, *Love Without End, Jesus Speaks...,* Heartwings, 1999.

Hay, Louise L., *You Can heal Your Life,* Hay House, 2004.

Hollingsworth, Elaine, *Take Control Of Your Health and Escape the Sickness Industry,* Empowerment Press International, 13th Edition.

Hunter, Beatrice Trum, *Additives Book, What You Need to Know,* Keats Publishing, Inc. Revised 1980.

Kloss, Jethro, *Back to Eden,* Woodbridge Press Publishing, original 1939, reprint 1975.

Life Science Publishers, *The People's Desk Reference for Essential Oils* Fourth Edition, 2009.

Marciniak, Barbara, *Bringers of the Dawn, Teachings from the Pleiadians,* Bear and Company Publishing 1992.

Nathan, Harold D., PhD, Henrickson, Charles, PhD, *CliffsQuickReview Chemistry,* Hungry Minds, 2001.

Nelson, William C. Prof., *Promorpheus: An Advanced Treatise in Subspace and Quantum Aspects of Biology,* The College of Practical Homeopathic, Reprint and edited 1996. http://www.downloads.imune.net/medicalbooks/The%20Promorpheus%20Treatise%20in%20Quantum%20Biology.pdf

Northrup, Christiane, M.D., *Women's Bodies, Women's Wisdom Creating Physical and Emotional Health and Healing,* Bantam Books, Revised 1998.

Overman, James R., ND, *Overcoming Parasites Naturally,*

234

Overman's Healthy Choices, Inc 2006

Pauling, Linus, *How to Live Longer and Feel Better,* W. H Freeman and Company 1986

Tolle, Eckhart, *The Power of Now,* New World Library, 1999

Venes, Donald, MD, MSJ Editor, *Taber's Cyclopedia Medical Dictionary Edition 22 Illustrated,* F.A. Davis, 2014.

Weisbar, Paul and Lillie, *Stillpoint Laser, Unwind and Dissolve Into Your Quantumfield,* Copyright 2011.

Young, Gary D., ND, *Essential Oils Integrative Medical Guide, Building Immunity, Increasing Longevity, and Enhancing Mental Performance with Therapeutic-Gade Essential Oils,* Essential Science Publishing 2003.

Notes

Preface

~ Alice Calaprice, collector and editor, The Ultimate Quotable Einstein, Princeton University Press and The Hebrew University of Jerusalem, 2011

Introduction

~ Calaprice, 187-188

1 Clayton L. Thomas, MD, M.P.H. Editor, *Taber's Cyclopedic Medical Dictionary, Edition 14 Illustrated,* (F.A. Davis Company), 1981. page 742, I-40.

2 Archives of Environmental Health: An International Journal, May/June 1999 issue, Vol. 54, No. 3, pp.147-149, April 2010, (Heldref Publications), *Multiple Chemical Sensitivity: A 1999 Consensus,* Dec 2012, http://www.heldref.org appears in the May/June 1999 issue (volume 54, number 3).

3 Center for Disease Control, *Leading Causes of Deaths: Final Data for 2013,* Feb 2015, www.cdc.gov/nchs/fastats/leading-cause-of-death.htm.

4 J. Eisenberg *Report to Congress on Research on Multiple Chemical Exposures and Veterans with Gulf War Illnesses.* Washington DC: US Department of Health and Human Services, Office of Public Health and Science. 15 January 1998, Sept 2014.

5 Research Advisory Committee on Gulf War Veterans' Illnesses, *Gulf War Illness and the Health of Gulf War Veterans: Research Update and Recommendations,* 2009-2013, 2015, Page 123.

6 Miriam-Webster.com, *Re-duc-tion-ism,* noun,
   1. explanation of complex life-science processes and phenomena in terms of the law of physics and chemistry; also; a theory or doctrine that complete

reductionism is possible

2. a procedure or theory that reduces complex data and phenomena to simple terms.

7   Desire Dubounet, *The Messenger Angel, The Messages of the Angel* The Science and Philosophy of Professor William Nelson (Change The World Productions, 2010) page 24.

"The two body problem is easily solvable. This has been used by science for hundreds of years. A ball falls to the earth, and we calculate the two forces and get a good result. But when there are three bodies (ball, earth, moon) it gets very difficult, but still solvable result. Science has struggled to reduce everything to the two body problem. This is called reductionism. So to test a drug they reduce the human to just one variable like blood pressure, give a drug and measure the change in blood pressure. Advanced science has learned that complex systems such as the human body are fractal in nature and reductionism fails, so they developed CHAOS theory. When more and more variables are measured we observe ... complex results. Things never repeat, and some small stimulus can have large effects. This is called the butterfly effect..."

8   Robert O. Becker, and Gary Seldon, *The Body Electric*, (William Morrow and Company, Inc.), 1985, page 230.

"None of our textbooks could tell us the how and why of healing. They explained the basics of scientific. They explained the basics of scientific medicine-anatomy, biochemistry, bacteriology, pathology, and physiology each dealing with one aspect of the human body and its discontents. Within each subject the body was further subdivided into systems. The chemistry of muscle and bone, for example was taught separately from that of the digestive tract and nervous systems. The same approach is used today, for fragmentation is the only way to deal with a complexity that would otherwise be overwhelming. The strategy works perfectly for understanding space ships, computes, or other complicated machines, and is very useful in biology. However, it leads to the reductionist assumption that once you understand the parts, you understand the whole. That approach ultimately fails in the study of living things-hence the widespread demand for an alternative, holistic medicine-for life is like no machine humans have ever built: It's always more than the sum of its parts."

CHAPTER ONE Experience is Knowledge: Reported Symptoms

~   Calaprice, 323

1   Merriam-Webster.com

2   Scott Whitaker, ND and Fleming, Jose, CN, *Medisin* (Divine Protection Publications, DPP, 326 West Hacienda Dr. Corona, CA 92882) Page 4.
     Defining "Cure" is when the observed symptoms from which the licensed professional deduced a "diagnosis" are no longer detectable and the patient is said to have been "cured" by the authorized "treatment" even if the patient dies several years later. For example, a patient is treated for a certain type of cancer with the application of chemotherapy, radiation, or surgery. The patient falls into a remission state for a couple of years, and then the cancer returns in another area of the body, but at an alarming rate the patients immune system is compromised even more as they succumb to death. and "Treat" is the process of providing drug material or other recognized medical treatments for the diagnosed "disease" or "condition." Most medical treatments such as hysterectomies, thyroid or gallbladder removal not only leaves the patient minus an important organ or gland, but the removal of a body function that will never be normal again.

3   FDA, *Glossary of Terms: Drugs, Feb 2012, Feb 2014,* www.fda.gov/drugs/informationondrugs/ucm079436.htm

4   Adrian Morris, MB, ChB, DCH, MFPG, *ABC of Allerogology,* Idiopathic Environmental Intolerance (IEI) Allergy Current Allergy and Clinical Immunology, March 2007 Vol 20, No.1.
     "Environmental Awareness" In the final analysis, after many

years of investigation, there appears to be no convincing evidence in the medical literature for the existence of MCS or EI. The underlying cause for the IEI symptom complex is unlikely to be a direct reaction to everyday chemicals, but rather a masked stress disorder with heightened olfactory awareness (hyperosmia) and associated unresolved psychological issues."

5   Carolyn Hax, *Dear Carolyn, Motherhood Alters Wife,* (Miami Herald) , February 26, 2015.

6   Heather Hansman, *The Newest Eating Disorder To (Maybe) Enter the DSM: Orthorexia,* (FastCompany.com), January 29, 2015.
"Orthorexia nervosa is a label designated to those who are concerned about eating healthy. Characterized by disordered eating fueled by a desire for "clean" or "healthy" foods, those diagnosed with the condition are overly pre-occupied with the nutritional makeup of what they eat". A push is on for inclusion in the Psychiatric Association's Diagnostic and statistical Manual of Mental Disorders or DSM.

7   *MTHFR*, Genetics Home Reference, Service of the U.S. National Library of Medicine, November 2014, October 2015. http://ghr.nlm.nih.gov/gene/MTHFR

8   Clayton, page 667, H-51. *Homeostasis* "State of equilibrium of the internal environment of the body that is maintained by dynamic processes of feedback and regulation. Homeostasis is dynamic equilibrium."

CHAPTER TWO Looking for a Cure in All the Wrong Places

~   Calaprice, 181

1   Andrew Anderson, *Pharmaceutical industry gets high on fat profits,* (BBC News) Nov 6, 2014, FEB 2015. www.bbc.news.com/news/business-28212223
"Last year five pharmaceutical companies made a profit

margin of 20% or more Pfizer, Hoffman-La Roche, AbbvVie, GlaxoSmithKline (GSK) and Eli Lily." "But as the table below shows drug companies spend far more on marketing drugs-in some cases twice as much- than on developing them. And beside, profit margins take into account R&D costs."

Pfizer
50.3 billion Total Revenue
6.6 billion spent on R&D
11.4 billion spent on Sales and Marketing
22.0 billion in Profits
43% Profit Margin

Hoffman-LaRoche
50.3 billion Total Revenue
9.3 billion spent R&D
9.0 billion in Sales and Marketing
12.0 Billion in Profit
24% Profit Margin

AbbVie
18.8 billion Total Revenue
2.9 billion spent in R&D
4.3 billion in Sales and Marketing
4.1 billion in Profits
22% Profit Margin

GlaxoSmithKline (GSK)
41.4 billion Total Revenue
5.3 billion spent in R&D
9.9 billion in Sales and Marketing
8.5 billion in Profits
21% Profit Margin

Eli Lily
23.1 billion Total Revenue
5.5 billion spent in R&D
5.7 billion in Sales and Marketing
4 billion in Profits
22% Profit Margin

Johnson & Johnson
71.3 billion Total Revenue
8.2 billion spent R&D,
17.5 billion Sales and Marketing,

13.8 billion Profit,
19% Profit Margin

2   Andrew Anderson, *Pharmaceutical industry gets high on fat profits*, (BBC News), Nov 6, 2014, FEB 2015. www.bbc.news.com/news/business-28212223
"Last year five pharmaceutical companies made a profit margin of 20% or more Pfizer, Hoffman-La Roche, AbbVie, GlaxoSmithKline (GSK) and Eli Lily"
BIG PHARMA FINES (Source:ProPublica)
$3 Billion Glaxo Smith Kline, 2012, over promoting PAXIL for depression to under age 18.
$2.3 Billion, Pfizer, 2009 over misbranding painkiller Bextra
$2.2 Billion Johnson & Johnson, 2013, for promoting drugs not approved as safe.
$1.42 Billion Eli Lily, 2009, for wrongly promoting anti-psychotic drug Zyprexa

3   U.S. Government Publishing Office, *Electronic Code of Federal Regulations, Part 182- Substances Generally Regarded As Safe,* Feb 2015, 2015,
www.ecfr.gov/cgi-bin/text-idx?
rgn+div5&node+21:3,0,1,1,13

4   Beatrice Trum Hunter, *Additives Book What You Need to Know*, (Keats Publishing), 1980page 115.
"The GRAS list must not be allowed to continue serving as a privileged status by exempting food additives from being adequately tested merely because they have been in long time use. Up to the present, the expenses for manufacturer. The FDA has brazenly proposed to transfer this financial burden to the taxpayer..... The cost of testing for profitable food chemicals must be borne by the food processors."

5   www.amgen.com, *Biologics, and Biosimilars an Overview*, April 2011, August 2015.

6   www.ars-grin.gov, *Dr. Duke's Phytochemical and Ethnobotanical Databases [online Database] 30 August 2015.*

7   Jeremy Rifkin, *The Hydrogen Economy*, Putnam/Jeremy P. Tarcher, http://encognitive.com/node/2183

8   CDC, *Workplace Safety and Health Topics: Known Carcinogen List*, May 2, 2012, Feb 2015. http://www.cdc.gov/niosh/topics/cancer/npotocca.html

9   http://www.bt.cdc.gov/agent/chlorine/basics/facts.asp

10 *The American Heritage® Science Dictionary.* "Trihalomethane." (Houghton Mifflin Company), 21 Feb.2015. Dictionary.com http://dictionary.reference.com/browse/trihalomethane

11 American Journal of Epidemiology, *Risk of Specific Birth Defects in Relation to Chlorination and the Amount of Natural Organic Matter in the Water Supply*, (John Hopkins Bloomberg School of Public Health), Vol. 156. No.4, April 2002, Feb 2015. page 374
    "Chlorination of drinking water that contains organic compounds leads to the formation of by-products, some of which have been shown to have mutagenic or carcinogenic effects" explain researchers led by Dr. Paul Magnus of the National Institute of Public Health in Oslo Norway. The findings suggest that "the risk of birth defects is highest in municipalities with both a high content of... organic compounds in drinking water and a practice of chlorination Magnus and colleagues conclude"

12 MS Malcom, P. Weinstein and AJ Woodward, *Something in the Water? A health impact assessment of disinfection by-products in New Zealand.* (PubMed.gov), US National Library of Medicine, National Institutes of Health, Oct 1999, Feb 2015. http://www.ncbi.nlm.nih.gov/pubmed/10606403 "Abstract"
    "The population attributable risk per cent, for cancers and birth defects in New Zealand, is about 25%. In other words, a quarter of all bladder, colon and rectal cancers and birth defects may be preventable by reducing DBP (disinfection by-products) exposure. This is equal to 329 preventable

cancer deaths in 1995 and 94 preventable birth defects in 1996. DBP exposure can be reduced without compromising microbiological safety of water supplies. The health effects of DBPs must be weighed against the cost of DBP reduction and not against the potential water borne disease prevented by disinfection."

13 Hunter, Page 97-100

CHAPTER THREE How Does Someone Get Like This?

~   Calaprice, 188

CHAPTER FOUR Trusting Nature

~   Calaprice, 95

CHAPTER FIVE The Earnest Endocrinologist

~   Calaprice, 180

1   My personal experience has been that the anxiety has happened as long as eight hours after the chemical exposure that triggered the anxiety response.

2   Christiane Northrup, M.D., *Women's Bodies, Women's Wisdom Creating Physical and Emotional health and Healing, Bantam Books*, Revised Edition 1998, Page 129

3   Wallach & Rubin, *The Pre-Menstrual Syndrome and Criminal Responsibility*, 19 UCLA L. Rev.209, 263 (1971-72).
http://heinonline.org/HOL/LandingPagecollection=journals &handle=hein.journals/wasbur24&div=13&id+&page
"On December 16, 1980, a thirty -six year old English woman ended a love affair by deliberately running down her lover with her car and killing him.(cited Regina v. English, an unreported decision by the Norwich Crown Court on November 10, 1981.). At trial she plead guilty to

manslaughter because of diminished responsibility (cited Diminished responsibility "permits a defendant charged with a crime which requires the accused to possess a specific intent to produce psychiatric testimony tending to show that because of some mental defect or disorder she or he did not have the state of mind required for conviction"

4   http://articles.baltimoresun.com/1991-06-16/news/19911
     67033_1_pms-richter-defense, (Newsday, June 16, 1991).
     "Judge Smith drew criticism from feminists fearful that a renaissance of old myths about "raging hormones" could deny women high level jobs or child custody. "This decision just gives ammunition to people who want to deny women particular jobs" said Shirley Sagawa of the National Women's Law Center"It reinforces the stereotypes that a lot of people have about PMS-that there is a certain time of the month when women become completely irrational and dangerous."

5   Hunter, Page 45,
     "severe allergic reactions have been reported for BHT (and BHA) including, "debilitating and disabling chronic asthmatic attacks," skin blistering, eye hemorrhaging, tingling sensations on face and hands, extreme weakness, fatigue, edema, chest tightness, and difficulty in breathing.

CHAPTER SIX The Mother Solvent

~   Calaprice, Page 384

1   Department of Health and Human Services, *Occupational Health Guideline for Toluene,* page 3 , Center for   Disease Control, September 1978, November 1981.
     Common Operations: Use as a solvent in pharmaceutical, chemical, rubber, and plastics industries; as a thinner for paints, lacquer, coatings, and dyes; as a paint remover; insecticides. Use as starting material and intermediate in organic chemical and chemical synthesis. Use in manufacture of artificial leather, fabric and paper coatings; photogravureink production; spray surface coating; as a

244

diluent. Use as constituent in formulation of automotive and aviation fuels.

2   U.S. Department of Health and Human Services, Public Health Services, Agency for Toxic Substances and Disease Registry, TOLUENE CAS#108-88-3 *What is Toluene?*, February 2001.
"Toluene is a clear, colorless liquid with a distinctive smell. Toluene occurs naturally in crude oil and in the tolu tree. It is also produced in the process of making gasoline and other fuels from crude oil and making coke from coal. Toluene is used in making paints, paint thinners, fingernail polish, lacquers, adhesives and rubber and in some printing and leather processes."

3   Merriam-Webster Dictionary, *Definition of Toluene,* March 2015. www.merriam-webster.com/dictionary/toluene

4   Scientific American Supplement, *The Estimation of Toluene in Crude Petroleum* ,Volume 84 Cornell University Library, Sage Endowment Fund Supplement No. 2172 , (Munn and Co. Inc, August 18, 1917) page 112.
"Since the war began the public has heard a great deal about benzene and toluene and aromatic hydrocarbons. The three chief aromatic hydrocarbons are benzene, toluene, and the three xylenes."

5   U.S. Geological Survey, *BTEX Definitions,* Department of the Interior, (Cohen and Mercer, 1993). June 2014 March 2015. www.toxics.usgs.gov/definitions/btex.html BTEX (benzene, toluene, ethylbenzene, and xylene) "Volatile, mono-cyclic aromatic compounds present in coal tar, petroleum products, and various organic chemical product formulations."

6   Office of Pollution Prevention and Toxics, *Chemicals in the Environment: Toluene (CAS No. 108-88-3),* August 1994, August 2012.
"Toluene (also called methyl Benzene) is a colorless, flammable liquid. It occurs naturally in petroleum crude oil.

Petroleum crude oil is by far the largest source of toluene. Most (up to a billion pounds each year) of this toluene is never isolated from crude oil. Refineries pump this "unrecovered" toluene to some other locations where it is added directly to gasoline. The toluene that is isolated is expected to grow moderately over the next several years. The largest users of "recovered" in large amounts (approx 800 million gallons in 1991) by twenty companies in the United States. US demand for toluene is expected to grow moderately over the next several years. The largest users of "recovered" toluene are companies that make benzene. Companies also add toluene to aerosol spray paints, wall paints, lacquers, paint strippers, adhesives, printing ink, spot removers, cosmetics, perfumes, and antifreeze.

7   Center for Disease Control, *Naphthas*, NIOSH Manual of Analytical Methods (NIMAMI), Fourth Edition, August 1994, March 2015.
    www.cdc.gov/niosh/docs/2003-154/pdfs/1550.pdf
    SYNONYMS: Petroleum ether (benzin, rubber solvent, petroleum naphtha, VM&P naphtha, mineral spirits, Stoddard solvent, kerosene (kerosine), coal tar naphtha

8   The Paleontological Research Institution, Petroleum Education The World of Oil, *Oil and Everyday Life*, Oct 2015.
    https://www.priweb.org/ed/pgws/uses/uses_home.html

9   Agency for Toxic Substances and Disease Registry, *Toluene*, Center for Disease Control, Sept 2000, updated January 21, 2015 ,March 2015.
    http://www.atsdr.cdc.gov/substances/toxsubstance.asp?toxid =29,

10 Canadian Centre for Occupational Health and Safety. *Toluene*. February 2013, March 2015.
    www.ccohs.ca/oshanswers/chemicals/chem_profiles/toluene. html
    Flammable Properties: HIGHLY FLAMMABLE LIQUID. Can ignite at room temperature. Releases vapor that can

form explosive mixture with air. Can be ignited by static discharge.

11 National Toxicology Program, *13th Report on Carcinogens (RoC0,* October 2014), March 2015,
http://ntp.niehs.nih.gov/go/roc13

12 Centers for Disease Control and Prevention, *Chemical Listing and Documentation of Revised IDLH Values,* l, December 14, 2014, March 6, 2015.
www.cdc.gov/niosh/idlh/intridl4.html#

13 www.users.rcn.com *Biology Papers, Parts Per Million,* March 3, 2011, August 3, 2015.

14 Agency for Toxic Substances and Disease Registry, *Public Heath Statement for Benzene,* Center for Disease Control, January 2015, February 2015.
http://www.atsdr.cdc.govphs/phs.asp?id=37&tid=14#

15 AFTSDR, page 6
http://www.atsdr.cdc.govphs/phs.asp?id=37&tid=14#

16 Environmental Protection Agency, Pre-publication Copy Notice: *Title: Proposed Rule -Toluene Diisocyanates (TDI) and Related Compounds; Significant New Use Rule* The Director of Pollution Prevention and Toxics: Federal Register document January 7, 2015), March 11 2015.
http://www.epa.gov/oppt/existingchemicals/pubs/actionplans/PrePubCopy_TDI%20SNUR_NPRM.pdf

17 Merriam-Webster Dictionary Definition of *Benzene* 2015, March 2015.
www.merriam-webster.com/dictionary/benzene

18 Agency for Toxic Substances and Disease Registry, *Benzene, (*Center for Disease Control, March 3, 2011), March 2015.
http://www.atsdr.cdc.gov/phs/phs.asp?id=37&tid=14
http://www.atsdr.cdc.gov/ToxProfiles/tp3-c1-b.pdf

19 www.essentialchemicalindustry.org,
    Benzene and Methylbenzenes, January 2, 2014, July 27, 2015

20 www.atsdr.cdc.gov, January 21, 2015, July 5, 2015

21 www.toxnet.nlm.nih.gov May 15, 2014, July 5, 2015

22 Wikipedia, *Feedstock and Example of Petrochemical Products*, Feb 2015.
    www.upload.wikimedia.org/wikipedia/commons/1/19/BTX-Derivatives.org
    Benzene feed stock examples of petrochemical products: Styrene, polystyrene, phenol, cumene, anline, adipic acid, nylons. Toluene feed stock examples of petrochemical products: benzolic acid, toluene diisocyanate, polyurethanes, caprolactam, nylons, polyureas

23 Harold D. Nathan, PhD, and Charles Henrickson, PhD., Cliffs Quick Review *Chemistry*, Hungry Minds, 2001, p.53.

24 www.chemed.chem.purdue.edu, *Structure and Nomenclature of Hydrocarbons.* June 2015.
    "What is an Organic Compound? 200 years Chemists have divided materials into two categories.
    Those isolated from plants and animals were classified as organic.
    Those isolated trace back to minerals were inorganic.
    "This is based on a once held belief that organic compounds were fundamentally different from the inorganic compounds because of a **vital force** that was found in living systems. The decline of vital force theory began in 1828 when Friederich Wohler synthesized urea from inorganic starting compounds. He was trying to make ammonium cyanate (NH4OCN) from silver cyanate (AgOCN) and ammonium chloride (NH4CI). What the end results of the organic synthesis of synthetic urea."

25 www.chem.sc.edu>shimizu>chem_333 "The valence electrons (VE) are the electrons in the outer shell of an atom..."

248

26 www.cs.stedwards.edu/.../scie2320_nutrition__outline_
    partII_rev2014- 07-21-28qjwz1.pdf
    St. Edwards's University, July 2015

27 BTEX Industry Visual (a) Petroleum distillation towers (b)
    Petroleum fractions March 6, 2015.
    www.chemwiki.ucdavis.edu/@api/deki/files/30452/07be65df
    beb661

28 Wikipedia, *Benzedrine,* Feb 2016.
    http://en.wikipedia.org/wiki/Benzodiazepin

29 US government, FDA, *Diethanolamine*, March 2013, March
    2015.
    www.fda.gov/cosmetics/ProductsIngredients/ucm109655.ht
    m

30 FDA, *Diethanolamine, March 2015.*

31 www.sciencelab.com, msds29.pdf, *Propylene glycol* MSDS,
    May 21, 2013, July 9 2015.

32 www.sciencelab.com msds28.pdf, *Sodium lauryl sulfate*
    MSDS, May 21, 2013, July 9, 2015.

33 www.sciencelab.com msds30.pdf, *tert-Butylhydroquinone*
    MSDS, May 21, 2013, July 9, 2015.

34 FDA, U.S. Government, *The FDA on the term NATURAL,*
    January, 2015, March, 2015.
    http://www.fda.gov/aboutfda/transparency/basics/ucm21486
    8.htm

35 www.shell.com, *Synthetic solvents,* "Unlike most
    hydrocarbon solvents, which are distillation 'cuts' from crude
    oil refining, Isoparaffins are synthesized (chemically made)
    through an alkylation process. Main applications: Paints and
    Coatings, Aerosol propellant, Extraction, Metalworking,
    Detergents, Cosmetics, Textile Cleaning.", July 2015.

36 Phil Lambert, *Food Q&A: Just what is 'natural' flavoring?*, (Today Food) April 7, 2004. October 2015.

37 Organic Consumers Association, *Organic Bytes: USDA Again Undermining Organic Integrity,* May 2004, March 2015.
https://www.organicconsumers.org/old_articles/bytes/06230 4.php

38 FDA, U.S. Government *Definition of Organic on food labels,* January 26, 2015, March 12, 2015.
http://www.fda.gov/AboutFDA/Transparency/Basics/ucm21 4869.htm,
"Q. Does FDA have a definition for the term "organic" on food labels?
A. No. The term "organic" is not defined by law or regulations FDA enforces."

39 USDA, U.S. Government, *The USDA defines term "organic".* June 2004, March 2015.
http://www.usda.gov/wps/portal/usda/usdahome/parentnav=F AQS_BYTOPIC&FAQ
NAVIGATION_ID=ORGANIC_FQ&FAQ_NAVIGATION_ TYPE=FAQS_BYTOPIC&contentid=faqdetail-3.xml&edeployment_action=retrievecontent

CHAPTER SEVEN A Quantum Turn of Events

~ Calaprice, page 230

CHAPTER EIGHT Death: The Final Symptom

~ Calaprice, page 435

1 http://www.imdb.com/name/nm0014877/

2 Rebecca Stone, *Today Tomorrow and Forever- In loving memory of Elvis Presley,* 2005, October2015
http://elvisforver.tripod.com/id3.html

CHAPTER NINE Leaf Me Forever

~   Calaprice, page 453

1   http://www.merriam-webster.com/dictionary/essential%20oil

2   http://www.iso.org/iso/home.html

3   http://www.afnor.org/en

4   Life Science Publishers, <u>Essential Oils Desk Reference</u>, <u>Fourth Edition</u>, Appendix P, *Comparative Antimicrobial Activity of Essential Oils and Antibiotics, January 2009.*

5   KA Hammer, CF Carson, TV Riley, *Antimicrobial activity of essential oils and other plant extracts.* Journal of Applied Microbiology, 1999,2015
    http://www.ncbi.nlm.nih.gov/pubmed/?term=10438227

6   Hulda Clark, <u>*The Cure and Prevention of All Cancers*</u>, (New Century Press, 1995) page 604.

CHAPTER TEN The Professor and a New Science

~   Calaprice, page 363

1   www.downloads.immune.net/medicalbooks/
    ThePromorpheusTreastiseQuantumBiology.pdf

2   Free Dictionary online *Promorphology*, noun.
    "Crystallography of organic forms;- a division of morphology created by Haeckel. It is essentially stereo metric, and relates to a mathematical conception of organic forms."

3   www.nlpu.com, *Neuro-linguistic programming* or NLP is a name that encompasses the three most influential components involved in producing human experience, neurology, language and programming.

4   Desire Dubounet, Electroceuticals, *The Thirty Year Development of Electroceuticals*,
http://medicalexposedownloads.com/PDF/The%2030%20ye ar%20Development%20of %20Electroceuticals.pdf

5   *Mind-Matter Interaction Research,* video Psyleron-Princeton, www.psyleron.com, May 23, 2015.
"**Narrator**: So can people affect machines with their minds?"
"**Brenda Dunne**: It would appear so. The Phenomenon are real. They aren't just due to chance effects. They're small occurrences. They don't seem to be associated with processes that we think of as cognitive. We don't see things like learning curves. We don't see any of the usual things associated with cognitive and psychological... It is if the probabilities are being changed rather the physical activity. We have seen:
     -Gender differences: independent of distance and time
     -Cooperative effect: appears with opposite sex emotionally bonded couples
     -Effects in groups: especially groups who are of the same wave length with an idea
All these are things challenging any attempt to model them because they don't fit with our prevailing   understanding with how the world works... The next level is, OK, the phenomenon is real."

6   Richard P. Feynman, *QED: The Strange Theory of Light and Matter*, (Princeton University Press) 1985.

7   Desire Dubounet, Professor of Medicine, *Electroceuticals*. May 2015 Reprinted with permission. Page 1
http://medicalexposedownloads.com/PDF/The%2030%20ye ar%20Development%20%20Electroceuticals.pdf

8   http://scienceforkids.kidipede.com/physics/electricity/ , May 2015. "Everything in the universe is made of atoms, and atoms are made of electricity. Atoms are made of even smaller particles called protons, neutrons, and electrons. The protons and neutrons (NOO-trons) are packed tightly

together in the middle of the atom, and we call them the nucleus (NOO-klee-uss) of the atom. Around the nucleus there are electrons, orbiting around and around the nucleus kind of the way that the earth goes around the sun. There's empty space between the electrons, so an atom is mainly empty space."

9   http://hyperphysics.phy-astr.gsu.edu ,
    Adenosine Triphosphate, June 2015.

10 http://en.wikipedia.org/wiki/Electrochemistry

11 Dubounet, page 45.

12 Nelson, *Promorpheus,* page 22
    "The theory of interaction of light with matter is called Quantum Electro Dynamics QED. Simply put, QED tells us that any minuscule quantum change in a part of matter will involve the release of absorption of a photon. When an electron absorbs a photon it jumps to a higher quantic state, When it releases the photon it jumps to a higher state . When it releases the photon it goes to a lower state. Also there are virtual particles, especially virtual photons, coming in and out of existence in the universe. The subject is made to appear more difficult than it actually is by the very much overly complex mathematics that constitutes the proof of the theory. One of the simplest is that of Fermi. We start by just postulating for the emission or absorption of photons."

13 Merriam-Webster Dictionary, *Covalent Bond,* "A covalent bond is defined as a chemical bond formed between atoms by the sharing of electrons."

14 www.hyperphysics.phy-astr.gus.edu, Aug 2015

15 Dubounet, p. 47

16 www.accessdata.fda.gov, Title 21, Volume 8, Cite: 21cfr 882.5050 revised as of April 1, 2014, June 4, 2015.
    "Sub Chapter H Medical Devices Biofeedback (a)

Identification. A biofeedback device is an instrument that provides a visual or auditory signal corresponding to the patient's physiological parameters (e.g. brain activity, skin temperature, etc.) so that the patient can control voluntarily these physiological parameters. (b) Classification. Class II (special controls) The device is exempt from the pre market notification procedures in sub part E of part 807 of this chapter when it is a prescription battery powered device that is indicated for relaxation training and muscle reeducation and prescription use."

17 www.wikipedia.com ,*Electrophysiological,* June 15, 2015, July 10, 2015

18 Merriam-Webster Dictionary, *quantum,* April 2015

19 www.fda.gov/AboutFDA/Transparency/Basics/ ucm194413.htm,
Does FDA regulate medical devices?, May 1, 2014, May 2015.

20 William Nelson, *"Nelsonian Medicine"*, as listed within the SCIO/EDUCTOR program reprinted with permission.

CHAPTER ELEVEN Living Proof: My Results

~ Calaprice, page 452

1 Http://www.stress.org.america-1-health-problem/

2 *Science and Spirituality TV, Interview of Dr. Fritz-Albert Popp,* YouTube.com, Part 1 video, Part 2 transcript, Published on Apr 27, 2014.

3 F.A. Popp, *New Adventures in Medicine.* Lectures: August-September 1979, Bioresonance and multiresonance therapy,ed. (Brugemann, Hans, Haug) International Vol.1.1993, p.175.

4 Hulda Clark, *Cure for all Diseases, (New Century Press,*

1995), Page 13. definition of "zapping is to selectively electrocute pathogens."

5   Steve Gamble,   THE DANGERS OF EMF RADIATION
AND WHAT WE CAN DO TO IMPROVE OUR HEALTH
IN TODAY'S POLLUTED WORLD *Can radiation from all electrical wiring, equipment, power lines, substations, and even battery operated items affect our biophysical and biological bodies, damage, alter our DNA and lead to illness and disease?, (www.Equilibrauk.com), July 2015.*

6   World Health Organization, International Agency for Research on Cancer, *IARC Classifies Radio frequency Electromagnetic Fields as Possibly Carcinogenic to Humans*, Press Release No. 208, May 31, 2011, Sept 5 2015.

7   Gamble

8   L. Hardell and C. Sage, *Biological effects from electromagnetic field exposure and public exposure standards,* Biomed Pharmacother, *(www.ncbi.nlm.nih.gov)*February 2008, July 2015.

CHAPTER TWELVE Pain Relief and a Nightlight!

~   Calaprice, page 388

1   Lily and Paul Weisbart, *Stillpoint Laser Unwind and Dissolve into your Quantumfield,* Copyright 2011 by Paul and Lily Weisbart.

2   Gamble, page 4

3   Pinar Avci, MD, Asheesh Gupta, PhD, and Michael R. Hamblin, PhD, *Low-level laser (light) therapy (LLLT) in skin: stimulating, healing,restoring,* www.ncbi.nlm.nih.gov, page 3.
Abstract: "The photons are absorbed by mitochondrial chromophores in skin cells. Consequently electron transport, adenosine triphosphate (ATP) nitric oxide release, blood

flow, reactive oxygen species increase and diverse signaling pathways get activated. Stem cells can be activated allowing increased tissue repair and healing."

4   Douglas Ashendorf, MD,. *Low Level Laser Therapy for Head, Neck and Facial Pain,* (FAAPMR, Newark, New Jersey The CFIDS Chronicle Physicians Forum Fall 1993) June 2015.
Prof P.F. Bradley: "The clinical application of low incident power density laser radiation for the treatment of acute and chronic pain is now a well established procedure. This paper reviews the currently available English speaking literature and summaries a selection of serious scientific papers which report a beneficial effect following the treatment of a wide variety of acute and chronic syndromes whose main presenting symptom is pain". Head and Neck Clinical Applications of LLLT is proving useful in a wide variety of painful conditions in the Head and Neck but the following are particular applications: 1. TM Joint Dysfunction 2. Post Herpetic Neuralgia 3. Trigeminal Neuralgia 4. Painful Ulcerative Conditions 5. Pain of Advanced Oro Facial Cancer. The ability of Low Level Light Therapy to Mitigate Fibromyalgia pain."

5   Pinar Avci, MD, Asheesh Gupta, PhD, and Michael R. Hamblin, PhD, *Low-level laser (light) therapy (LLLT) in skin: stimulating, healing , restoring ,*
www.ncbi.nlm.nih.gov, page 3.
Abstract: "The photons are absorbed by mitochondrial chromophores in skin cells. Consequently electron transport, adenosine triphosphate (ATP) nitric oxide release, blood flow, reactive oxygen species increase and diverse signaling pathways get activated. Stem cells can be activated allowing increased tissue repair and healing."

6   Nicholas West, *The 10 Inventions of Nicola Tesla that Changed the World,* (www.bibliotecapleyades.net), Jan 5, 2012, July 17, 2015.
"Upon Tesla's death on January 7, 1943, the U.S. Government moved into his lab and apartment confiscating

all of his scientific research, and to this day none of his research has been made public.

The Ten Inventions:

1. Alternating Current
2. Light tubes, florescent light
3. X-Rays
4. Radio
5. Remote Control
6. Electric Motor
7. Robotics
8. Laser
9. Wireless Communications
10. Limitless Free Energy"

7   Dubounet, page 11

8   Weisbart, page 28

9   Weisbart, page 18

10 P. Rola, A. Doroszko,   and A.Derkacz , *The Use of Low Level Energy Laser Radiation in Basic and Clinical Research, (www.ncbi.nlm.nih.gov,),* Sept 2014, July 2015.

11 F. Gonzalez-Lima and Douglas W. Barret, *Augmentation of Cognitive Brain Functions with Transcranial Lasers,* www.ncbi.nim.nih.gov.

12 Segen's Medical Dictionary, *Cold laser,* (Farlex, Inc.) 2012. "A hand-held, nonsurgical laser using photobiostimulation, which received FDA approval for treating carpal tunnel syndrome. Benefits claimed for cold lasers include increased collagen production, nerve regeneration, bone and tissue repair, vasodilation, enzyme response, cell metabolism, cell membrane potential, pain threshold, and reduced inflammatory duration and oedema."

13 VN Koshelev and Iu V Chalyk, *The causes of fatalities in liver and spleen injuries, (www.ncbi.nim.nih.gov),* July 2015. (Article in Russian) "Abstract: The authors have analyzed

results of treatment of 170 patients with traumas of the liver and 129 patients with injuries of the spleen. It was established that the leading factors responsible for lethaltities were severity of shock, blood loss volume, and the amount of associated injuries. The authors have shown that laser coagulation for hemostasis could reduce the amount of lethaltities and gave less amount of post operative complications."

14 Hulda Clark, *A Cure for All Diseases,* (New Century Press) Reprinted 2007, page 251

15 Hulda Clark, page 36-37

CHAPTER THIRTEEN The Anti-Steroid

~ Calaprice, page 273

CHAPTER FOURTEEN Travelers on a Less Traveled Road

~ Calaprice, page 451, paraphrased

1 Stephanie Hampton , Monsanto Discredited Bureau Swings into Action, March 27, 2015, April 2015 www.dailykos.com/story/2015/3/27/1373484/-monsanto-s-discredit-bureau-swings-into-action.by   occupystephanie "Recently I attended a talk by Monsanto's Dr. William "Bill" Moar who presented the latest project in their product pipeline dealing with RNA. Most notably, he also spoke about Monsanto's efforts to educate citizens of their genetically engineered products. The audience was mostly agricultural students many of whom were perhaps hoping for the only well-paid internships and jobs in their field. One student asked what Monsanto was doing to counter the "bad science" around their work. Dr. Moar, perhaps forgetting that this was a public event, then revealed that Monsanto indeed had *"an entire department"* (waving his arm for emphasis) dedicated to *"debunking"* science which disagreed with theirs. As far as I know this is the first time that a Monsanto functionary has publicly admitted that they have such an

entity which brings their immense political and financial weight to bear on scientists who dare publish against them. The Discredit Bureau will not be found on their official website."

2   Jeffery Smith, *GMO Researchers Attacked, Evidence Denied, and a Population at Risk*, Sept 19, 2012/April 2015. www.GlobalResearch.com
"Early 1990s Dr. Arpad Pusztai, Biologist had more than 300 articles and 12 books to his credit and was the world's top expert in his field. But when he accidentally discovered that genetically modified foods are dangerous, he became bio-tech industry's bad boy poster child. Dr. Arpad Pusztai saw his career ruined by big government and big agribusiness because he told the truth about GMO good. Employed by Rowett Institute in Aberdeen Scotland for 35 years. Awarded $3 million grant by UK government to design a system for safety testing of GM food. Within ten days of feeding rats GM potatoes the animals developed potentially pre-cancer cell growth, smaller brains, livers, testicles, and partially atrophied livers and damaged immune systems. Moreover the cause was almost certainly side effects from the process of genetic engineering itself."

3   Danell Glade, *List of over 100 Dead Microbiologists*, Feb 20, 2016/Apr 18, 2016.
http://prepareforchange.net/2016/02/20/list-of-over-100-dead-microbiologists/
"The worlds top anti-virus microbiologists are being killed off. By 2005, 40 were dead. Today, over 100. Many murdered, the rest died under very suspicious circumstances. It is known they were all working on highly sensitive or government-funded research projects tied to bio-weapons and viral pandemic. Are these silenced 'whistle blowers' who knew too much? Why didn't the mainstream media report in on these stories?"

CHAPTER FIFTEEN MSDS: Material Safety Data Sheets

~ Calaprice, page 303

1 National Institute for Occupational Safety and Health, *NIOSH Pocket Guide To Chemical Hazards, Toluene,* (Department of Heath and Human Services Sept 2005), Centers for Disease Control and Prevention, page 311. FI.P 40' F, class 1B Flammable liquid

2 Agency for Toxic Substances and Disease Registry, *Toxicological Profile for Toluene,* (U. S. Department of Health and Human Services September 2000), March 2015, Page 177. Toluene is listed as a toxic substance under Section 313 of the emergency Planning and Community Right to Know Act (EPCRA) under Title III of the Superfund Amendments and Reauthorization Act (SARA) (EPA 1995j). www.atsdr.cdc.gov/toxprofiles/tp56.pdf

3 Google: *Define permeator:* A permeator is a chemical which can pass through the outer protective dermal layers and into the body, and can either expose the body to toxic effects of that chemical or act as a carrier for other toxic/hazardous chemicals.

4 *IARC's Report on Glyphosate, (www.monsanto.com/IARCreportonGlyphosate),* July 20, 2015. "IARC concluded that glyphosate belongs in a 2A category that includes professions such as barbers and fry cooks. The 2A classification does not establish a link between glyphosate and an increase in cancer. "Probable " does not mean that glyphosate causes cancer and IARC's conclusion conflicts with the overwhelming consensus"

5 International Agency for Research on Cancer, *IARC Monographs Volume 112: evaluation of five organophosphate insecticides and herbicides,* (World Health Organization) March 20, 2015. page 1-2 "For the herbicide glyphosate, there was limited evidence of

carcinogenicity in humans for non-Hodgkin lymphoma. The evidence in humans is from studies of exposure, mostly agricultural, in the USA, Canada, and Sweden published since 2001. In addition, there is convincing evidence that glyphosate also can cause cancer in laboratory animals. On the basis of tumors in mice, the United States Environmental Protection Agency originally classified glyphosate as *possibly carcinogenic to humans* in 1985. After a re-evaluation of that mouse study, the US EPA changed its classification to evidence of *non-carcinogenicity in humans (Group E)* in 1991. The US EPA advisory Panel noted that the re-evaluated glyphosate results were still significant using two statistical test recommended in the IARC Preamble. The IARC Working Group that conducted the evaluation considered the significant findings from the US EPA report and several more recent positive results in concluding that there is Sufficient evidence of carcinogenicity in experimental animals. Glyphosate also caused DNA and chromosomal damage in human cells, although it gave negative results in tests using bacteria. One study in community residents reported increases in blood markers of chromosomal damage (micronuclei) after glyphosate formulations were sprayed nearby.

How are people exposed to these pesticides?

Glyphosate currently has the highest global production volume of all herbicides. The largest use worldwide is in agriculture. The agricultural use of glyphosate has increased sharply since the development of crops that have been genetically modified to make them resistant to glyphosate. Glyphosate is also used in forestry, urban, and home applications. Glyphosate has been detected in the air during spraying, in water, and in food. The general population is exposed primarily through residence near sprayed areas, home use and diet, and the level that has been observed is generally low.

What do Groups 2A... mean?

Group 2A means that the agent is *probably carcinogenic to humans*. This category is used when there is limited evidence of carcinogenicity in humans and sufficient evidence of carcinogenicity in experimental animals. *Limited evidence* means that a positive association has been observed between exposure to the agent and cancer but that other explanations for the observations (called chance, bias, or confounding) could not be ruled out. This category is also used when there is limited evidence of carcinogenicity in humans and strong data on how the agent causes cancer.

How were the evaluations conducted?

The established procedures for Monographs evaluations is Described in the Programs Preamble. Evaluations are performed by panels of international experts, selected on the basis of their expertise and the absence of real or apparent conflicts of interest. For Volume 112, a Working Group of 17 experts from 11 countries met at IARC on 3-10 March 2015 to assess the carcinogenicity of tetrachlorvinphos, parathion, malathion, diazinon, and glyphosate. The in-person meeting followed nearly a year of review and preparation by the IARC secretariat and the Working Group, including a comprehensive review of the latest available scientific evidence. According to published procedures, the Working Group considered "reports that have been published or accepted for publication in the openly available scientific literature" as well as "data from governmental reports that are publicly available: The working group did not consider summary tables in online supplements to published article, which did not provide enough detail for independent assessment."

6   PMEP Pesticide Management Education Program, *Glyphosate - Chemical Profile 2/85,* (Cornell University Cooperative Extension, New York State, 2/7/1985) March 10, 2015.
http://pmep.cce.cornell.edu/profiles/herb-growthreg/fatty-alcohol-monuron/glyphosate/glyphos_prf_0285.html.
"There are no specific antidotes for these chemicals. Because manifestations of toxicity do occasionally occur in peculiarly predisposed individuals..."

CHAPTER SIXTEEN Resources

~   Calaprice, page 17

BIBLIOGRAPHY

~ Calaprice, page 425

Made in United States
North Haven, CT
14 February 2023

32586669R00153